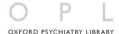

O P L

OXFORD PSYCHIATRY LIBRARY

# Obsessive-Compulsive
# and Related Disorders

D1614381

O   P   L
OXFORD PSYCHIATRY LIBRARY

# Obsessive-Compulsive and Related Disorders

## Second Edition

## Doctor Samar Reghunandanan

Consultant Psychiatrist, Department of Psychiatry, North Essex partnership
University NHS Foundation Trust, Essex and Honorary Research Psychiatrist,
Highly Specialized Obsessive Compulsive and Related Disorders Service,
Hertfordshire Partnership NHS University Foundation Trust, Welwyn Garden
City, Hertfordshire, UK

## Visiting Professor Naomi A. Fineberg

Consultant Psychiatrist, Highly Specialized Obsessive Compulsive and Related
Disorders Service, Hertfordshire Partnership University NHS Foundation
Trust, Welwyn Garden City, Hertfordshire and Professor, Postgraduate
Medical School, University of Hertfordshire, College Lane, Hatfield, UK

## Professor Dan J. Stein

Professor, Department of Psychiatry,
University of Cape Town, and
Director, Medical Research Council Unit on
Anxiety & Stress Disorders, South Africa

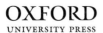

OXFORD
UNIVERSITY PRESS

# OXFORD
### UNIVERSITY PRESS

Great Clarendon Street, Oxford, OX2 6DP,
United Kingdom

Oxford University Press is a department of the University of Oxford.
It furthers the University's objective of excellence in research, scholarship,
and education by publishing worldwide. Oxford is a registered trade mark of
Oxford University Press in the UK and in certain other countries

First Edition published in 2007
Second Edition published in 2015

Impression: 1

Published in the United States of America by Oxford University Press
198 Madison Avenue, New York, NY 10016, United States of America

British Library Cataloguing in Publication Data

Data available

Library of Congress Control Number: 2015938201

ISBN 978–0–19–870687–8 (pbk.)

Printed and bound in Great Britian by
Clays Ltd, St Ives plc

Oxford University Press makes no representation, express or implied, that the
drug dosages in this book are correct. Readers must therefore always check
the product information and clinical procedures with the most up-to-date
published product information and data sheets provided by the manufacturers
and the most recent codes of conduct and safety regulations. The authors and
the publishers do not accept responsibility or legal liability for any errors in the
text or for the misuse or misapplication of material in this work. Except where
otherwise stated, drug dosages and recommendations are for the non-pregnant
adult who is not breast-feeding

Links to third party websites are provided by Oxford in good faith and
for information only. Oxford disclaims any responsibility for the materials
contained in any third party website referenced in this work.

# Contents

# Abbreviations

| | |
|---|---|
| ACC | anterior cingulate cortex |
| ACT | acceptance and commitment therapy |
| ADHD | attention deficit hyperactivity disorder |
| ArKO | aromatase knockout |
| BAP | British Association for Psychopharmacology |
| BDD | body dysmorphic disorder |
| CBT | cognitive behavioural therapy |
| CGI | Clinical Global Impression |
| COMT | catechol-O-methyltransferase |
| CR | controlled-release |
| CRT | cognitive remediation therapy |
| CSF | cerebrospinal fluid |
| CSTC | cortico-striatal-thalamic-cortical |
| CY-BOCS | Children's Yale–Brown Obsessive Compulsive Scale |
| DA | dopamine |
| DBS | deep brain stimulation |
| DSM | Diagnostic and Statistical Manual |
| DY-BOCS | Dimensional Yale–Brown Obsessive Compulsive Scale |
| ECA | Epidemiological Catchment Area |
| ECG | electrocardiogram |
| ECT | electro convulsive therapy |
| ERP | exposure and response prevention |
| GABA | gamma aminobutyric acid |
| GP | general practitioner |
| 5-HIAA | 5-hydroxy-indoleacetic acid |
| HIV | human immunodeficiency virus |
| 5-HT | serotonin |
| ICD | International Classification of Disease |
| INR | international normalized ratio |
| MAOA | monoamine oxidase A |
| mCPP | *m*-chloro-phenylpiperazine |
| mg | milligram |
| MINI | Mini International Neuropsychiatric Interview |
| mL | millilitre |

| | |
|---|---|
| MRI | magnetic resonance imaging |
| MRS | magnetic resonance spectroscopy |
| ng | nanogram |
| NICE | National Institute for Health and Care Excellence |
| NNH | number needed to harm |
| NNT | number needed to treat |
| OCD | obsessive-compulsive disorder |
| OCDs | obsessive-compulsive and related (spectrum) disorders |
| OCRDs | obsessive-compulsive related disorders |
| OFC | orbitofrontal cortex |
| PANDAS | paediatric autoimmune neuropsychiatric disorder associated with streptococcal infections |
| PET | positron emission tomography |
| PFC | prefrontal complex |
| RCT | randomized controlled trial |
| rTMS | repetitive transcranial magnetic stimulation |
| SERT | serotonin transporter |
| SRI | serotonin reuptake inhibitor |
| SSRI | selective serotonin reuptake inhibitor |
| TNF | tumour necrosis factor |
| VMPFC | ventromedial prefrontal cortex |
| VMS | ventromedial striatum |
| WFSBP | World Federation of Societies for Biological Psychiatry |
| WHO | World Health Organization |
| Y-BOCS | Yale–Brown Obsessive Compulsive Scale |
| Z-FOCS | Zohar–Fineberg Obsessive Compulsive Screen |

# Chapter 1

# Introduction

There are several reasons for thinking that obsessive-compulsive disorder (OCD) is one of the most important conditions in psychiatry.

First, epidemiological evidence has indicated that OCD may be one of the most prevalent and disabling of the psychiatric disorders (Karno et al. 1988). Indeed, it is remarkable to note that, in early data from a seminal World Health Organization (WHO) study of the burden of disease, OCD was characterized as one of the most disabling of all medical disorders (Murray and Lopez 1996). Although there remains some debate about the exact prevalence of OCD, there is no question that this condition is extremely costly, not only in terms of individual and family suffering (Amir et al. 2000; Fineberg et al. 2013), but also in terms of cost to society (Hollander et al. 1997). A consideration of the obsessive-compulsive and related (spectrum) disorders (OCDs), rather than just OCD, further expands the magnitude of the problem.

Second, OCD arguably comprises a paradigmatic exemplar of a neuropsychiatric disorder. It is a relatively homogeneous disorder, with studies consistently revealing an association with particular neurocircuitry (cortico-striatal-thalamic-cortical, CSTC) and specific neurotransmitter systems (e.g. serotonin) (Fineberg et al. 2014; Stein 2002). Recent advances in OCD include molecular imaging studies of specific receptors, whole genome association studies, and the identification of endophenotypes. Although there may be important environmental contributors to OCD, the early view of OCD as caused by psychogenic conflict can no longer be supported (Stein and Stone 1997).

Third, OCD and obsessive-compulsive related disorders (OCRDs) provide clinician-scientists, and others interested in translational research, with a unique opportunity to develop an integrated cognitive–affective neuroscience approach to psychiatric disorder. OCD was not only one of the first disorders shown in controlled studies to respond to both pharmacotherapy and psychotherapy, it was also the first condition in which both treatment modalities were demonstrated to normalize the underlying functional neuroanatomy. The growing set of animal, genetic, and molecular imaging studies of OCD, taken together with rigorous work on the phenomenology and neurocircuitry of OCD and OCRDs, provide a unique opportunity for scientists to develop translation models of obsessive-compulsive psychopathology and to move between bench and bedside in studying its treatment.

Fourth, there is now an extensive database of randomized controlled trials of treatment of OCD, allowing for an evidence-based approach to its management. This database covers both pharmacotherapy and psychotherapy, both first-line and augmentation trials, both acute and long-term studies, and studies in both adults and children (Fineberg et al. 2012). Professional organizations have drawn on this extensive database, in order to develop high-quality guidelines and algorithms for the treatment of OCD and OCRDs. Consumer organizations have been able to encourage people suffering from symptoms to establish an early diagnosis and to receive appropriate treatment. Although additional work is needed to move the investigation of OCD and OCRDs from studies of efficacy to those of effectiveness in real-world settings, there is already an important opportunity to take knowledge from randomized controlled trials and to apply it in everyday practice.

Taken together, the results of this broad-based programme of research have strengthened the conceptualization of OCD and OCRDs as disabling mental disorders, characterized by the inability to flexibly control stereotyped and repetitive cognitive and behavioural responses. This was recognized in the recent fifth revision of the American Psychiatric Association *Diagnostic and Statistical Manual* (DSM-5, 2013) where OCD is now grouped within a new Obsessive-Compulsive and Related Disorders chapter, together with body dysmorphic disorder (BDD), hoarding disorder, trichotillomania (hair-pulling disorder), and excoriation (skin-picking) disorder. It is hoped that this reclassification will generate new avenues of research into the psychobiological mechanisms governing adaptive and pathological aspects of compulsivity that will drive forward new treatments for this disabling group of disorders.

In this volume, we aim to summarize the phenomenology, pathogenesis, pharmacotherapy, and psychotherapy of the OCRDs, focusing on OCD as the exemplar disorder for which the majority of the scientific data is available. Many reviews exist in the academic literature of each of these areas. The aim of the current volume is to synthesize the findings in a succinct and practical way, in order that it is as useful as possible for clinicians, and hopefully therefore also for patients suffering from OCRDs.

# References

American Psychiatric Association (APA). (2013). *Diagnostic and Statistical Manual of Mental Disorders*, 5th edition *(DSM-5)*. Washington, DC: APA.

Amir N, Freshman M, and Foa EB (2000). Family distress and involvement in relatives of obsessive–compulsive disorder patients. *J Anxiety Disord*. **14**: 209–17.

Fineberg NA, Brown, A, Reghunandanan S, and Pampaloni I. (2012). Evidence-based pharmacotherapy of obsessive–compulsive disorder. *Int J Neuropsychopharmacol*. **9**: 1–19.

Fineberg NA, *et al*.; Obsessive Compulsive and Related Disorders Research Network. (2013). Manifesto for a European research network into obsessive–compulsive and related disorders. *Eur Neuropsychopharmacol*. **23**: 561–8.

Fineberg NA, *et al*. (2014). New developments in human neurocognition: clinical, genetic, and brain imaging correlates of impulsivity and compulsivity. *CNS Spectr*. **19**: 69–89.

Hollander E, *et al*. (1997). A pharmacoeconomic and quality of life study of obsessive–compulsive disorder. *CNS Spectr*. **2**: 16–25.

Karno M, *et al*. (1988). The epidemiology of obsessive–compulsive disorder in five US communities. *Arch Gen Psychiatry*. **45**: 1094–9.

Murray CJL and Lopez AD. (1996). *Global Burden of Disease: A Comprehensive Assessment of Mortality and Morbidity from Diseases, Injuries and Risk Factors in 1990 and Projected to 2020*, Vol. I. Harvard: World Health Organization.

Stein DJ. (2002). Seminar on obsessive–compulsive disorder. *Lancet*. **360**: 397–405.

Stein DJ and Stone MH. (1997). *Essential Papers on Obsessive–Compulsive Disorders*. New York: New York University Press.

# Chapter 2

# Phenomenology

## Key points

- OCD and OCRDs are common lifespan illnesses that cause substantial suffering.
- Patients may hide symptoms, and OCD and OCRDs are frequently overlooked by health professionals.
- Direct enquiry about OCD and OCRDs can help accurately identify these conditions.
- Factor analyses consistently identify particular symptom clusters in OCD.
- Measures for screening, diagnosis, and assessing OCD and OCRDs symptom severity are available.

## 2.1 Symptoms

OCD is characterized by intrusive, unpleasant thoughts or images (obsessions), and by repetitive, unwanted actions (compulsions) that the individual feels driven to perform in response to obsessions or according to rigid rules. Although obsessions typically increase anxiety, they are not simply real-life worries. The consequent compulsions may serve to decrease or increase anxiety. The diagnostic criteria for OCD in the *Diagnostic and Statistical Manual of Mental Disorders* (DSM-5) (American Psychiatric Association 2013) emphasize that compulsions can be either observable behaviours or mental rituals. While patients typically recognize the excessiveness of their symptoms, there is a range of insight, and some may be classified as suffering from the 'poor insight' or 'absent insight/delusional' subtypes.

A broad range of possible obsessions and compulsions may be found. The commonest involve concerns about contamination with consequent washing, or concerns about harm to self or others with consequent checking. Factor analysis has demonstrated additional sub-groups involving symptom clusters such as symmetry concerns and arranging rituals, hoarding, and collecting (Bloch et al. 2008) (Table 2.1). Other common OCD symptoms include sexual, religious, somatic, and musical obsessions (Stein et al. 2001a). Individuals with hoarding appear less responsive to conventional treatment (Stein et al. 2008), and indeed hoarding symptoms that are unrelated to classical obsessions and compulsions have been reclassified in the DSM-5 (American Psychiatric Association 2013) as a separate, stand-alone disorder—hoarding disorder.

While predominant symptoms may alter for an individual over time (Swedo et al. 1989), the constancy of OCD symptomatology across time (pathological scrupulosity, for example) and place (similar symptoms occur across many cultures) is striking (Stein and Rapoport 1996). Moreover, symptoms in children and adults appear remarkably similar, although they may reflect the developmental level; for example, young children may have more concrete kinds of rituals.

| Table 2.1 OCD symptom clusters | |
|---|---|
| Obsessions | Compulsions |
| Contamination concerns | Washing, bathing, showering |
| Harm to self/others, sexual/religious concerns | Checking, praying, asking for reassurance |
| Symmetry, precision concerns | Arranging, ordering |
| Completeness concerns/inability to discard | Collecting/hoarding |

Symptoms differ, to some degree, in patients with and without tics (Jaisoorya et al. 2008). Patients with a current or past history of tic disorder may be more responsive to antipsychotic augmentation of serotonin reuptake inhibitors (SRIs) than those without tics (Phillips et al. 2010), perhaps pointing to underlying biological differences (see Chapter 3). Patients with obsessional slowness may also have another form of OCD that is characterized by a greater degree of neurological impairment (Veale 1993).

Overall, only minimal changes were made to the DSM-IV diagnostic criteria for OCD (American Psychiatric Association 1994) in the DSM-5. However, two substantive changes were made to specifiers: 1) addition of a specifier for the presence/history of tic disorder and 2) expansion of the poor insight specifier to include good or fair insight, poor insight, and absent insight/delusional OCD beliefs (to aid the differentiation of OCD from psychotic disorders). The next edition of the World Health Organization's International Classification of Disease (ICD-11) diagnostic guidelines are likely to be broadly consistent with the DSM-5.

## 2.2 **Obsessive-compulsive and related disorders**

The inclusion of a separate chapter within the DSM-5 devoted to OCRDs (American Psychiatric Association 2013; Phillips et al. 2010), which includes body dysmorphic disorder (BDD), hoarding disorder, trichotillomania (hair-pulling disorder), and excoriation (skin-picking) disorder, reflects both the increasing strength of evidence supporting these disorders' interrelatedness, in terms of diagnostic validators, **and** the clinical utility of grouping them together. Like OCD, these OCRDs are characterized by repetitive, unwanted obsessions/preoccupations or behaviours/mental acts, together with attempts to restrain the behaviours. Clinicians are encouraged to screen for each of these disorders in individuals presenting with an OCRD, in view of the high rates of shared comorbidity (Lochner and Stein 2010). Nonetheless, there remain important differences in diagnostic validators and treatment approaches across these disorders, as well as close relationships between some of the OCRDs and various other categories, including the anxiety disorders and the eating disorders (e.g. OCD, BDD) (Stein et al. 2010).

In several OCRDs, symptoms are focused around aspects of the self or one's body. BDD is characterized by a preoccupation with perceived defects in physical appearance that are either not visible or appear as minor flaws to others. BDD is associated with repetitive checking, neutralizing behaviours or mental acts, and a high level of social avoidance. Trichotillomania is characterized by repeated, distressing hair pulling with attempts to resist or stop this behaviour. It is similar, in some ways, to excoriation (skin-picking) disorder, which is characterized by repeated picking of one's skin, resulting in skin lesions, and repeated attempts to reduce or stop skin picking. Hoarding disorder is characterized by a persistent difficulty with discarding possessions, regardless of their actual value, either due to a strong need to save, or distress associated with discarding, possessions.

Several other putative OCD spectrum disorders are not included in the DSM-5 chapter on OCRDs. These include Tourette's disorder, which is classified as neurodevelopmental disorder in the DSM-5, and hypochondriasis, which is included in the DSM-5 as illness anxiety disorder. Obsessive-compulsive personality disorder is characterized by an enduring and maladaptive pattern of excessive perfectionism and rigidity, need for control, and overconscientiousness. While obsessive-compulsive personality disorder continues to be classified as a personality disorder in DSM-5, consideration is being given to including it both with OCRDs and personality disorders in ICD-11.

## 2.3 **Diagnostic threshold**

By definition, OCD symptoms are accompanied by marked distress and dysfunction; this is the standard clinical significance criterion in the DSM classification (Spitzer and Wakefield 1999). Subclinical obsessive-compulsive symptoms are fairly common in the general population (Fineberg et al. 2013a) and are certainly seen during the course of normal development. In patients with OCD, however, it is usually not difficult to appreciate the tremendous suffering associated with this condition. Indeed, many studies have documented that quality of life in OCD is severely affected (Hollander et al. 2010; Stein et al. 2000).

## 2.4 **Differential diagnosis**

OCRDs should be differentiated from obsessive-compulsive syndromes resulting from a general medical disorder or ingestion of a substance (DSM-5). As discussed in more detail (see Section 2.8) obsessive-compulsive symptoms may be seen in a range of neurological disorders involving CSTC circuits; they may emerge after the administration of dopamine agonists (such as methylphenidate or cocaine), and occasionally during treatment with second-generation antipsychotics such as clozapine (Schirmbeck and Zink 2013).

Despite occasional overlap, OCD symptoms differ clearly from the fears and worries seen in other anxiety disorders, from the depressive ruminations characteristic of mood disorders and from the delusions of psychotic disorders. A number of other mental disorders, not so far classified as OCRDs, share aspects of obsessive-compulsive phenomenology, which can lead to particular diagnostic uncertainty. For example, as noted in Section 2.2, the obsessions and compulsions that characterize OCD need to be differentiated from the inflexible character traits that constitute obsessive-compulsive personality disorder, such as perfectionism, need for control, and overconscientiousness. In addition, OCD should not be confused with the repeated preoccupation about imagined illness and reassurance seeking that constitutes hypochondriasis. Eating disorders, such as anorexia nervosa, for which the focus is maintaining a low body weight, involve obsessive preoccupation with body size and shape and eating patterns and should be distinguished from BDD and obsessive-compulsive personality disorder.

Obsessive-compulsive symptoms also comprise an intrinsic component of a number of neuropsychiatric conditions, including autistic spectrum disorders, characterized by motor stereotypies, rigidity, and inflexibility manifested as a narrow behavioural repertoire and need for sameness; and Tourette's syndrome, characterized by repetitive, sudden, and rapid non-rhythmic motor movement or vocalization; and frontal lobe lesions.

## 2.5 **Prevalence**

The Epidemiological Catchment Area (ECA) studies provided the first epidemiological data on OCD that were based on a nationally representative sample and reliable diagnostic criteria. OCD was found to be the fourth most prevalent psychiatric disorder, with a lifetime prevalence of 2.5% (Karno *et al.* 1988). A cross-national study employing similar methodology demonstrated somewhat similar prevalence rates across a range of different populations (Weissman *et al.* 1994). A review of community studies suggested that, despite some concerns about the validity of the diagnosis of OCD in the ECA studies (Nelson and Rice 1997), OCD is common in both adult (Bebbington 1998) and paediatric (Zohar 1999) populations, with many studies yielding prevalence estimates along the lines of those found by the ECA investigators (Fineberg *et al.* 2013a; Kessler *et al.* 2005; Ruscio *et al.* 2010; Wittchen and Jacobi 2005). A recent community-based study found that around 20% of the general population reported a subclinical level of obsessive-compulsive symptomatology (Fineberg *et al.* 2013a).

The male to female ratio of OCD is roughly similar, particularly in clinical settings, in contrast to many other anxiety and mood disorders, in which the prevalence in females is higher. Age of onset in OCD may have a bimodal distribution. A subset of patients has onset at puberty or earlier; juvenile-onset OCD may be particularly common in males and appears to have other distinguishing characteristics such as greater familiality and relationship to tic disorders (Phillips *et al.* 2010). In a longitudinal community-based study, around two-thirds of OCD cases had emerged by the age of 22 years, and no new cases developed OCD after around 37 years (Fineberg *et al.* 2013a). Patients with a later onset include those developing OCD after pregnancy, miscarriage, or parturition (Rosso *et al.* 2012).

## 2.6 Comorbidity

Epidemiological studies are consistent with clinical work, showing a substantial lifetime comorbidity of OCD with other mental disorders, including depression, which developed in approximately two-thirds of cases presenting for treatment, specific phobia (22%), social phobia (18%), eating disorder (17%), alcohol dependence (14%), panic disorder (12%), and Tourette's syndrome (7%) (Pigott *et al.* 1994). A significant association with bipolar disorder has also been identified (Fineberg *et al.* 2013b). There is also substantial comorbidity within the OCRDs (Phillips *et al.* 2010). Most forms of comorbidity increase distress and impact negatively on family and work relationships, though disorder-specific effects have been observed. Thus, agoraphobia and generalized anxiety disorder have been found to be associated with increased OCD severity, bipolar disorder with suicidal acts, and panic disorder with increased treatment-seeking behaviour (Fineberg *et al.* 2013b). A subgroup of OCD patients may have impulsive features, including childhood conduct disorder symptoms, attentional deficits, and an increased rate of suicide attempts (Masi *et al.* 2006).

## 2.7 Course and burden of illness

Although acute episodes of OCD have been documented (Ravizza *et al.* 1996), and considerable variability exists in the periodicity, duration, and severity of illness, OCD, as seen in the psychiatric clinic, is usually a chronic disorder (Marcks *et al.* 2011; Pinto *et al.* 2006), and complete recovery is not commonly reported (Skoog and Skoog 1999), though cases are likely to show improvements over time. Intermittent episodes of OCD are thought to occur more frequently in the early stages of illness, and those with an early episodic course may experience a better long-term prognosis (Skoog and Skoog 1999). In non-clinical cohorts, the course of OCD may be more variable (Angst *et al.* 2004). In a recent analysis of a community-based cohort, followed up prospectively over 30 years, more than three-quarters of individuals with clinically relevant obsessive-compulsive syndromes entered a sustained period of remission to the extent that half of all cases had OCD for no more than 5 years and three-quarters had OCD for no more than 7 years consecutively. Individuals with a longer duration of illness, greater number of obsessive-compulsive burdened years, and those seeking professional help experienced significantly delayed remission. In addition, these factors, together with male gender and comorbid affective disorder, were associated with significantly reduced remission rates (Fineberg et al. 2013c).

OCD is associated with significant direct and indirect costs (Dupont et al. 1995; Lopez and Murray 1998). These are compounded by a lack of recognition, underdiagnosis, and inappropriate treatment. Patients may be too embarrassed to visit a clinician or may not be aware that help is available; the lag time from symptom onset to correct diagnosis was 17 years in one survey (Hollander et al. 1997). Preliminary results suggest that, as in the case of schizophrenia, a longer duration of untreated OCD is associated with poorer treatment outcomes (dell'Osso et al. 2010). The World Health Organization recently ranked OCD within the 20 leading causes of medical disability. The socio-economic costs associated with untreated OCD, estimated in one American study as 6% of the total cost associated with mental illness (Dupont et al. 1995), are substantial. Cost-effective therapies that can be offered in primary or secondary medical care settings are being developed. Better recognition and treatment of the disorder is now starting to be recognized by government health departments as a major public health objective (e.g. <http://www.nice.org.uk>).

## 2.8 **Obsessive-compulsive disorder in the non-psychiatric setting**

Given that patients may not describe their symptoms to clinicians (Newth and Rachman 2001), it is important to be aware of the possible presentation of OCD in a range of psychiatric and non-psychiatric medical settings (Fineberg et al. 2008). In dermatology clinics, for example, washing rituals may be common. Patients asking for cosmetic surgery may suffer from somatic obsessions, and patients in general medical clinics from hypochondriacal obsessions; neurology patients with involuntary movement disorders (Tourette's syndrome, Sydenham's chorea, Huntington's disorder) may have comorbid OCD; paediatric patients may have OCD after streptoccocal infection, and pregnant patients may experience de novo or increased OCD symptoms either during pregnancy or after delivery. Table 2.2 shows just some of the common areas where OCD patients present for treatment.

| Table 2.2 Presentations for treatment | |
|---|---|
| Professional | Reason for consultation |
| General practitioner (GP) | Depression, anxiety |
| Dermatologist | Chapped hands, eczema, trichotillomania |
| Cosmetic surgeon | Concerns about appearance (BDD) |
| Oncologist | Fear of cancer |
| Urologist | Fear of human immunodeficiency virus (HIV) |
| Neurologist | OCD associated with Tourette's syndrome |
| Obstetrician | OCD during pregnancy or the puerperium |
| Gynaecologist | Vaginal discomfort from douching |

> **Box 2.1 Zohar–Fineberg Obsessive Compulsive Screen (Z-FOCS): five screening questions for OCD**
>
> 1. Do you wash or clean a lot?
> 2. Do you check things a lot?
> 3. Is there any thought that keeps bothering you that you would like to get rid of but can't?
> 4. Do your daily activities take a long time to finish?
> 5. Are you concerned about orderliness or symmetry?
>
> © Joseph Zohar and Naomi A. Fineberg, 2006.

## 2.9 **Awareness and screening**

Despite growing awareness, many doctors and nurses have not been trained to detect OCD. Given patients' possible reluctance about disclosure, it is important for clinicians to ask the right questions. Although it can take years before individuals find a health professional in whom they can confide, direct enquiry by a sympathetic health practitioner is usually successful. Arguably, practitioners in areas known to attract large numbers of patients need to be primed to look for characteristic symptoms and enquire proactively, using targeted questions (Fineberg *et al.* 2008). Mental health workers should consider incorporating a form of 'brief screening' into every mental state examination (Heyman *et al.* 2006).

The Zohar–Fineberg Obsessive Compulsive Screen (Z-FOCS) (Box 2.1) was originally devised by J Zohar for the International Council on OCD. It consists of five simple questions designed to be administered by a doctor or a nurse and takes less than 1 minute to administer (Fineberg and Roberts 2001). A positive response to any of the questions should lead to detailed enquiry for OCD.

## 2.10 **Assessment**

Evaluation of OCD requires a thorough psychiatric history and examination to assess OCD symptoms and comorbid disorders, and to allow a differential diagnosis from other anxiety, mood, and psychotic disorders. A general medical history and examination should also be obtained. In some patients, OCD symptoms begin in the aftermath of infection (Swedo *et al.* 1998). Comorbid tics are not uncommon but are often overlooked, and patients should be carefully observed for them, as they may signal a different treatment pathway. Similarly, children with OCD should be asked about problems with attention and concentration, since attention deficit hyperactivity disorder (ADHD) may easily be missed. Indications for special investigations, such as structural brain imaging, might include late-onset symptoms, atypical symptoms, or severe treatment refractoriness.

Although the diagnosis is usually confirmed by a clinical interview, the use of brief standardized interviews, such as the Mini International Neuropsychiatric Interview (MINI) (Sheehan *et al.* 1994), for diagnosis may be useful. It may also be helpful to inquire about the patient's own explanatory model of their disorder—their theories of its cause and treatment. Patients with scrupulosity, for example, may see their symptoms in religious terms (Ciarrochi 1995). Some patients adhere to a view that unresolved, unconscious conflict is a cause of symptoms, and others that lack of self-confidence or fears of losing control are responsible. Being aware of these models and offering alternative perspectives are key steps in starting treatment. Consumer advocacy groups (Stein *et al.* 2001b) and Internet virtual groups (Stein 1997) may usefully contribute to such psycho-education (see Chapter 6).

People with OCD are sometimes poor at gauging their level of impairment, particularly during treatment when they may have difficulty recognizing signs of improvement. It can be helpful to ask a family member to corroborate the patient's history. The Yale–Brown Obsessive Compulsive Scale (Y-BOCS) (Goodman *et al.* 1989) measures the severity of OCD. It is sufficiently user-friendly to be easily administered in clinical practice, and its reliability and validity and sensitivity to change have made it the current 'gold standard' in OCD RCTs. The scale has also been adapted for use in children and adolescents (see Appendices 1 and 2: Y-BOCS and CY-BOCS, respectively), and for assessment of OCD spectrum disorders such as BDD. The Dimensional Y-BOCS (DY-BOCS) extends the Y-BOCS to allow evaluation of OCD severity, according to current dimensional models of OCD and symptom clusters (see Appendix 3: DY-BOCS). The Clinical Global Impression Severity and Improvement Scales (Guy 1976) are rapid measures of global severity and improvement that have been well validated for OCD and shown to be sensitive to change in treatment trials. There are also structured diagnostic interviews (du Toit *et al.* 2001) and self-rating scales (Le Beaut *et al.* 2013) available for the OCRDs.

# References

American Psychiatric Association. (1994). *Diagnostic and Statistical Manual of Mental Disorders*, 4th edn. Washington, DC: American Psychiatric Press.

American Psychiatric Association (APA). (2013). *Diagnostic and Statistical Manual of Mental Disorders*, 5th edn (*DSM-5*). Washington, DC: APA.

Angst J, et al. (2004). Obsessive–compulsive severity spectrum in the community: prevalence, comorbidity, and course. *Eur Arch Psychiatry Clin Neurosci.* **254**: 156–64.

Bebbington PE. (1998). Epidemiology of obsessive–compulsive disorder. *Br J Psychiatry.* **Suppl 35**: 2–6.

Bloch MH, et al. (2008). Meta-analysis of the symptom structure of obsessive–compulsive disorder. *Am J Psychiatry.* **165**: 1532–42.

Ciarrocchi JW. (1995). *The Doubting Disease: Help for Scrupulosity and Religious Compulsions.* Mahwah, NJ: Paulist Press.

Dell'Osso B, Buoli M, Hollander E, and Altamura AC (2010). Duration of untreated illness as a predictor of treatment response and remission in obsessive–compulsive disorder. *World J Biol Psychiatry.* **11**: 59–65.

Dupont RL, et al. (1995). Economic costs of obsessive–compulsive disorder. *Med Interface.* **8**: 102–9.

du Toit PL, et al. (2001). Comparison of OCD patients with and OCD patients without comorbid putative obsessive–compulsive spectrum disorders using a structured clinical interview. *Compr Psychiatry.* **42**: 291–300.

Fineberg NA and Roberts A. (2001). Obsessive compulsive disorder: a twenty-first century perspective. In: Fineberg NA, Marazitti D, Stein D, eds. *Obsessive Compulsive Disorder: A Practical Guide.* London: Martin Dunitz.

Fineberg NA, et al. (2008). Clinical screening for obsessive–compulsive and related disorders. *Isr J Psychiatry Rel Sci.* **45**: 151–60.

Fineberg NA, et al. (2013a). A prospective population-based cohort study of the prevalence, incidence and impact of obsessive–compulsive symptomatology. *Int J Psychiatry Clin Pract.* **17**: 170–8.

Fineberg NA, et al. (2013b). Lifetime comorbidity of obsessive–compulsive disorder and sub-threshold obsessive–compulsive symptomatology in the community: impact, prevalence, socio-demographic and clinical characteristics. *Int J Psychiatry Clin Pract.* **17**: 188–96.

Fineberg NA, et al. (2013c). Remission of obsessive–compulsive disorders and syndromes; evidence from a prospective community cohort study over thirty years. *Int J Psychiatry Clin Pract.* **17**: 179–87.

Goodman WK, et al. (1989). The Yale–Brown Obsessive Compulsive Scale. I. Development, use, and reliability. *Arch Gen Psychiatry.* **46**: 1006–11.

Guy W. (1976). *ECDEU Assessment Manual for Psychopharmacology, revised. US Dept Health, Education, and Welfare publication (ADM) 76–338.* Rockville, MD: National Institute of Mental Health.

Heyman I, et al. (2006). Obsessive–compulsive disorder. *BMJ.* **333**: 424–9.

Hollander E, *et al.* (1997). A pharmacoeconomic and quality of life study of obsessive–compulsive disorder. *CNS Spectr.* **2**: 16–25.

Hollander E, *et al.* (2010). Quality of life outcomes in patients with obsessive–compulsive disorder: relationship to treatment response and symptom relapse. *J Clin Psychiatry.* **71**: 784–92.

Jaisoorya TS, *et al.* (2008). Obsessive–compulsive disorder with and without tics—a comparative study from India. *CNS Spectr.* **13**: 705–11.

Karno M, *et al.* (1988). The epidemiology of obsessive compulsive disorder in five US communities. *Arch Gen Psychiatry.* **45**: 1094–9.

Kessler RC, *et al.* (2005). Lifetime prevalence and age of onset distribution of DSM-IV disorders in the National Comorbidity Survey Replication. *Arch Gen Psychiatry.* **62**: 593–602.

LeBeau RT, *et al.* (2013). Preliminary assessment of obsessive–compulsive spectrum disorder scales for DSM-5. *J Obs Compuls Rel Disord.* **2**: 114–18.

Lochner C and Stein DJ. (2010). Obsessive–compulsive spectrum disorders in obsessive–compulsive disorder and other anxiety disorders. *Psychopath.* **43**: 389–96.

Lopez AD and Murray CCJL. (1998). The global burden of disease, 1990–2020. *Nat Med.* **4**: 1241–3.

Marcks BA, *et al.* (2011). Longitudinal course of obsessive–compulsive disorder in patients with anxiety disorders: a 15 year prospective follow-up study. *Compr Psychiatry.* **52**: 670–7.

Masi G, *et al.* (2006). Comorbidity of obsessive–compulsive disorder and attention deficit disorder in reffered children and adolescents. *Compr Psychiatry.* **47**: 42–7.

Nelson E and Rice J. (1997). Stability of diagnosis of obsessive–compulsive disorder in the Epidemiologic Catchment Area study. *Am J Psychiatry.* **154**: 826–31.

Newth S and Rachman S. (2001). The concealment of obsessions. *Behav Res Ther.* **39**: 457–64.

Phillips KA, *et al.* (2010). Should an obsessive–compulsive spectrum grouping of disorders be included in DSM-V? *Depress Anxiety.* **27**: 528–55.

Pigott TA, *et al.* (1994). Obsessive compulsive disorder: comorbid conditions. *J Clin Psychiatry.* **55**(Suppl): 15–27; discussion 28–32.

Pinto A, *et al.* (2006). The Brown Longitudinal Obsessive Compulsive Study: clinical features and symptoms of the sample at intake. *J Clin Psychiatry.* **67**: 703–11.

Ravizza L, *et al.* (1996). Drug treatment of obsessive–compulsive disorder (OCD): long-term trial with clomipramine and selective serotonin reuptake inhibitors (SSRIs). *Psychopharmacol Bull.* **32**: 167–73.

Rosso G, *et al.* (2012). Obsessive–compulsive disorder during pregnancy and post-partum. *Riv Psichiatr.* **47**: 200–4.

Ruscio AM, *et al.* (2010). The epidemiology of obsessive–compulsive disorder in the National Comorbidity Survey: replication. *Mol Psychiatry.* **15**: 53–63.

Schirmbeck F and Zink M. (2013). Comorbid obsessive–compulsive symptoms in schizophrenia: contributions of pharmacological and genetic factors. *Front Pharmacol.* **4**: 99.

Sheehan DV, *et al.* (1994). *Mini International Neuropsychiatric Interview (MINI).* Tampa, FL: University of South Florida Institute for Research in Psychiatry; and Paris: INSERM—Hôpital de la Salpetrière.

Skoog G and Skoog I. (1999). A 40-year follow-up of patients with obsessive–compulsive disorder. *Arch Gen Psychiatry.* **56**: 121–7.

Spitzer RL and Wakefield JC. (1999). DSM-IV diagnostic criterion for clinical significance: does it help solve the false positive problem? Am J Psychiatry. **156**: 1856–64.

Stein DJ. (1997). Psychiatry on the internet: survey of an OCD mailing list. *Psychiat Bull.* **21**: 95–8.

Stein DJ and Rapoport JL. (1996). Cross-cultural studies and obsessive–compulsive disorder. *CNS Spectr.* **1**: 42–6.

Stein DJ, *et al.* (2000). Quality of life in obsessive–compulsive disorder. *CNS Spectr.* **5**(Suppl 4): 37–9.

Stein DJ, *et al.* (2001a). Unusual symptoms of OCD. In: Fineberg N, Marazziti D, Stein DJ, eds. *Obsessive Compulsive Disorder: A Practical Guide.* London: Martin Dunitz, pp. 37–50.

Stein DJ, *et al.* (2001b). Value and effectiveness of consumer advocacy groups: a survey of the anxiety disorders support group in South Africa. *Depress Anxiety.* **13**: 105–7.

Stein DJ, *et al.* (2008). Escitalopram in obsessive–compulsive disorder: response of symptom dimensions to pharmacotherapy. *CNS Spectr.* **13**: 492–8.

Stein DJ, et al. (2010). Should OCD be classified as an Anxiety Disorder in DSM-V? Depress Anxiety. **27**: 495–506.

Swedo S, et al. (1989). Cerebral glucose metabolism in childhood onset obsessive–compulsive disorder. Arch Gen Psychiatry. **46**: 518–23.

Swedo SE, et al. (1998). Pediatric autoimmune neuropsychiatric disorders associated with streptococcal infections: clinical description of the first 50 cases. Am J Psychiatry. **155**: 264–71.

Veale D. (1993). Classification and treatment of obsessional slowness. Br J Psychiatry. **162**: 198–203.

Weissman MM, et al. (1994). The cross national epidemiology of obsessive compulsive disorder. J Clin Psychiatry. **55**(Suppl): 5–10.

Wittchen HU and Jacobi F. (2005). Size and burden of mental disorder in Europe: a critical review and appraisal of 27 studies. Eur Neuropsychopharmacol. **15**: 357–76.

Zohar AH. (1999). The epidemiology of obsessive–compulsive disorder in children and adolescents. Child Adolesc Psychiatr Clin North Am. **8**: 445–60.

# Further reading

Fineberg NA, et al. (2013a). A prospective based cohort study of the prevalence, incidence and impact of obsessive–compulsive symptomatology. Int J Psychiatry Clin Pract. **17**: 70–8.

Fineberg NA, et al. (2013b). Lifetime comorbidity of obsessive–compulsive disorder and sub-threshold obsessive–compulsive symptomatology in the community: impact, prevalence, socio-demographic and clinical characteristics. Int J Psychiatry Clin Pract. **17**: 88–96.

Fineberg NA, et al. (2013c). Remission of obsessive–compulsive disorders and syndromes; evidence from a prospective community cohort study over thirty years. Int J Psychiatry Clin Pract. **17**: 79–87.

Skoog G and Skoog I. (1999). A 40-year follow-up of patients with obsessive–compulsive disorder. Arch Gen Psychiatry. **56**: 121–7

Williams KE and Koran LM. (1997). Obsessive–compulsive disorder in pregnancy, the puerperium, and the premenstruum. J Clin Psychiatry. **58**: 330–4.

# Chapter 3

# Pathogenesis

## Key points

- CSTC neurocircuitry plays a key role in OCRDs.
- Serotonin (5-HT), dopamine, (DA), and glutamate receptors in CSTC circuits appear particularly important.
- Particular variations in 5-HT, DA, and glutamate genes may contribute to vulnerability to OCD.
- Immune mechanisms may also play a role in contributing to CTSC dysfunction.
- OCD may involve a failure to inhibit evolutionarily-based procedural strategies.
- Both pharmacotherapy (SSRIs) and psychotherapy (cognitive behavioural therapy, CBT) can reverse CSTC dysfunction.

## 3.1 Introduction

In this chapter, we review the current understanding of the pathogenesis of OCRDs, focusing on OCD, as this disorder has been best studied. Whereas OCD was once primarily conceptualized as a psychogenic disorder, it is now increasingly conceptualized as a neuropsychiatric condition, mediated by a specific neurocircuitry. As we understand more about the cognitive and affective phenomena mediated by the neuronal abnormalities in these disorders and as we learn about the genes and proteins which mediate these neuronal changes, so an integrated cognitive–affective neuroscience of OCRDs becomes possible.

## 3.2 Neuroanatomy

Perhaps the earliest indication that OCD is mediated by specific neuronal circuits came from work showing an association between post-encephalitis parkinsonian and obsessive-compulsive symptoms occurring together with striatal lesions (Cheyette and Cummings 1995). OCD symptoms occurring in a range of other neurological disorders with striatal involvement, including Tourette's syndrome, Sydenham's chorea, Huntington's disorder, and Parkinson's disorder, were also documented by early authors (Stein et al. 1994) (Table 3.1). Such findings have been confirmed in a range of more recent systematic investigations.

Conversely, OCD patients have been found to demonstrate abnormalities in a broad series of measures and paradigms used in neuropsychiatric (e.g. neurological soft signs, olfactory identification, evoked potentials, prepulse inhibition, intracortical inhibition) and neuropsychological (e.g. executive function, visual memory function) research (Fineberg et al. 2010; Purcell et al. 1998a; Stein et al. 1994). These neuropsychiatric and neuropsychological abnormalities have consistently pointed to CSTC dysfunction and impaired control of the inhibition of thoughts and behaviours (Morein-Zamir et al. 2010), and some evidence has suggested that they are relatively specific to OCD (Purcell et al. 1998b) and disorders characterized by compulsive behaviours (Chamberlain and Menzies 2009; Fineberg et al. 2014; Phillips et al. 2010).

| Table 3.1 Lesions of the basal ganglia associated with OCD | |
|---|---|
| Infectious/immune | Post-encephalitic parkinsonism, Sydenham's chorea |
| Traumatic/toxic | Head injury, wasp sting, manganese intoxication |
| Vascular/hypoxic | Infarction, carbon monoxide intoxication, neonatal hypoxia |
| Genetic/idiopathic | Tourette's syndrome, Huntington's disease, neuroacanthocytosis |

Reproduced from *Current Insights in Obsessive Compulsive Disorder*, Edited by E. Hollander, J. Zohar, D. Marazziti, and B. Olivier, Copyright (1994), with permission from John Wiley and Sons.

Robust evidence from cognitive studies in OCD suggests deficits exist in aspects of flexible responding, impulse control, habit learning, and executive planning, thought to result from aberrant tuning of the CSTC circuits (Chamberlain *et al.* 2005; Gillan *et al.* 2014; Menzies *et al.* 2008). The finding of shared abnormalities in unaffected first-degree relatives of OCD probands for some of these changes suggests that these are trait deficits representing intermediate endophenotypes, otherwise called endophenotypes that mediate family-based illness vulnerability. Overlapping abnormalities have been observed in trichotillomania, skin-picking disorder, and BDD (reviewed in Fineberg *et al.* 2014), suggesting OCD-related endophenotypes cross diagnostic boundaries. Characterization of these changes is helpful to: (a) provide a more sophisticated account of the OCD phenotype than is offered by psychiatric criteria alone and (b) provide the link between clinical phenomena and brain imaging data.

Advances in brain imaging have provided the most persuasive neuroanatomic data on OCD (Menzies *et al.* 2007; Rauch and Baxter 1998; Whiteside *et al.* 2004). Structural imaging has pointed, in a number of studies, to abnormalities such as decreased volume or increased grey matter density in CSTC circuits (reviewed in Fineberg *et al.* 2010). Reduced cortical grey matter volume, coupled with increased basal ganglia grey matter volume, was found to correlate with neurocognitive indices of increased motor disinhibition in a study of OCD families (Menzies *et al.* 2007). This finding is consistent with theories implicating reduced top–down cortical control of striatally mediated behaviours as a pathogenetic mechanism in OCD. Discrepancies in structural imaging studies exist (de Wit *et al.* 2014), however, and may partly reflect the heterogeneity of OCD; for example, patients with OCD secondary to streptococcal infection (see Section 3.6) may have increased striatal volumes (Giedd *et al.* 2000), whereas patients with more chronic illness may have decreased volumes.

Functional imaging has consistently found that OCD is characterized by increased activity in areas (mainly medial) within the orbitofrontal cortex (OFC), cingulate, and striatum at rest and especially during exposure to feared stimuli (Figure 3.1). Somewhat different circuits may be involved in mediating the different OCD symptom clusters (Mataix-Cols *et al.* 2005; Saxena *et al.* 2004). The use of sophisticated cognitive and affective paradigms has confirmed the involvement of CSTC circuits in OCD (Chamberlain *et al.* 2008; Rauch *et al.* 2001); for example, during implicit learning, OCD subjects do not show the expected increase in striatal activity but instead employ more temporal cortical regions (Rauch *et al.* 2001). Interestingly, OCD subjects and unaffected relatives exhibited reduced orbitofrontal activation during a reversal learning challenge that correlated with reduced activation in the lateral OFC (Chamberlain *et al.* 2008) The observation that some behavioural challenges, such as exposure to OCD cues, induce over-activation of the OFC, and others under-activation, on functional imaging may be explained by functional segregation within the OFC.

The application of molecular imaging methods to OCD is at an early stage (Benazon *et al.* 2003; Denys *et al.* 2004; Rosenberg *et al.* 2001; Talbot 2004; van der Wee *et al.* 2004) but supports the structural and functional findings. Thus, magnetic resonance spectroscopy (MRS) demonstrated alterations in glutamate and glutamine in the CSTC circuits in OCD (Rosenberg

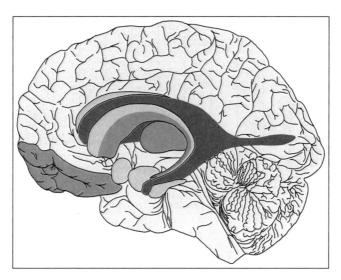

**Figure 3.1** Increased activity in the orbitofrontal cortex, ventral striatum, and thalamus in OCD. (Reproduced with permission of the University of Stellenbosch.)

*et al.* 2004; Whiteside *et al.* 2006; Yucel *et al.* 2008), and in some cases these alterations normalized after successful treatment with an SSRI (Rosenberg *et al.* 2000), while studies of dopaminergic receptors in the striatum have also demonstrated abnormalities (Denys *et al.* 2013).

Other regions of the brain have less commonly been suggested to play a role in OCD. For example, temporal dysfunction has occasionally been associated with OCD (Hugo *et al.* 1999; Zungu-Dirwayi *et al.* 1999), and there is some evidence of amygdala involvement (Szeszko *et al.* 1999). The supramarginal gyrus, supplementary motor cortex, and parietal lobe play a major role in the initiation and flexible control of instrumental behaviour and have also been implicated in brain imaging studies (Chamberlain *et al.* 2008; Meunier *et al.* 2012). Paediatric imaging research has supported the involvement of CTSC circuits in OCD and potentially offers the promise of being able to determine the evolution of brain abnormalities in different regions over time (Rosenberg and Keshavan 1998; Rosenberg *et al.* 2000).

Remarkably, both successful pharmacotherapy and behavioural therapy are able to normalize activity in CSTC circuits (Baxter *et al.* 1992) (Figure 3.2). It is notable that OCD was the first disorder in which studies of this kind were done, and subsequent analogous work in other disorders has contributed to an integrated view of the mind–body. Interestingly, baseline structure or activity may differentially predict response to pharmacotherapy and psychotherapy (Brody *et al.* 1998; Hoexter *et al.* 2013), so that different modalities may be effective via different mechanisms.

Neurosurgical interruption of CSTC circuits may also reduce symptoms (Jenike 1998; Rauch *et al.* 2004) and decrease striatal volume (Rauch *et al.* 2000). Deep brain stimulation, a new surgical treatment which involves the implantation of electrodes to chronically stimulate nodes within the CSTC circuitry, has been shown to normalize electrical activity and reduce connectivity within the CSTC circuits during symptom provocation in patients with OCD (Bourne *et al.* 2012).

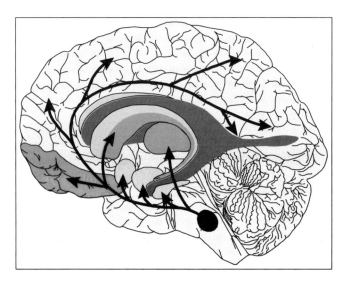

**Figure 3.2** Normalization of CSTC circuits by either pharmacotherapy or psychotherapy in OCD. The black arrows represent the serotonergic neurons originating in the raphe and projecting widely to CSTC and other regions. (Reproduced with permission of the University of Stellenbosch.)

## 3.3 Neurocognition

A new perspective on the role of CSTC circuitry in the pathophysiology of OCRDs has been derived from recent research into compulsivity and impulsivity. These neuropsychological domains involve dissociable cognitive functions, mediated by neuroanatomically and neurochemically distinct components of the cortico-subcortical circuitry. The constructs were historically viewed as diametrically opposed, with impulsivity being associated with risk seeking and compulsivity with harm avoidance. However, they are increasingly recognized to be linked by shared neuropsychological mechanisms involving dysfunctional inhibition of thoughts and behaviours.

Traditionally, compulsive disorders, such as OCD and BDD, and impulsive disorders, such as pathological gambling and possibly trichotillomania, were viewed at opposite ends of a single dimension, the former driven by a desire to avoid harm and the latter by reward-seeking behaviour. Again, convergent evidence from translational studies now suggests that a shared tendency toward behavioural disinhibition, presumably resulting from failures in 'top–down' cortical control of fronto-striatal circuits, or alternatively from overactivity within the striatal circuitry, may crucially underpin both compulsive and impulsive disorders. Thus, rather than polar opposites, compulsivity and impulsivity may represent key orthogonal factors that each contribute, to varying degrees, across these disorders (Fineberg *et al.* 2010).

The OCRDs represent a group of mental disorders for which both compulsive and impulsive behaviours appear, at least on phenotypic grounds, to be the core and most damaging ingredient. By exploring these pathologies, using tasks of cognitive performance that tap into these specific functions and/or by functional imaging studies that measure activity within these neural systems, new neuroanatomical models are under development. These models posit the existence of separate, but intercommunicating, 'compulsive' and 'impulsive' cortico-striatal circuits, differentially modulated by neurotransmitters (Brewer and Potenza 2008; Robbins 2007).

In the compulsive circuit, a dorsal striatal component (caudate nucleus) may drive compulsive behaviours, and a prefrontal component (OFC) may exert inhibitory control over them. Similarly, in the impulsive circuit, a ventral striatal component (ventral striatum/nucleus accumbens shell) may drive reward-focused impulsive behaviours, and a prefrontal component (anterior cingulate cortex (ACC)/ventromedial prefrontal cortex (VMPFC)) may exert inhibitory control. In disorders characterized by motor impulsivity, such as hair-pulling disorder, the right inferior frontal cortex and its connections to the globus pallidus may play an analogous role. Thus, in this model, there exist at least two striatal neural circuitries (dorsal compulsive, ventral impulsive) that drive these behaviours, and two corresponding prefrontal circuitries that restrain these behaviours. Hyperactivity within the striatal components or abnormalities (presumably hypoactivity) in the prefrontal components may thus result in an increased automatic tendency for executing either impulsive or compulsive behaviours, depending on the sub-component afflicted (Figure 3.3). Anatomical overlap between these functional systems, so that what starts out as a problem in the impulsive circuit may end up as a problem in the compulsive circuit and vice versa, may explain the impulsive–compulsive diathesis model for obsessive-compulsive and related disorders (Hollander and Wong 1995).

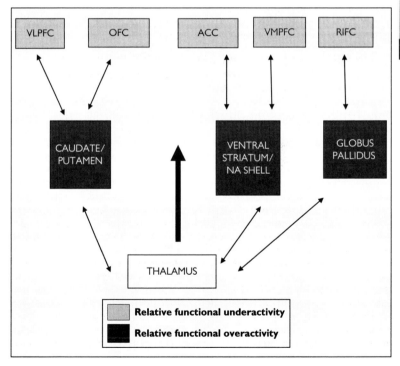

**Figure 3.3** Theoretical model of the compulsive and impulsive CSTC circuits simplified. Although impulsive and compulsive disorders can be envisaged as polar opposites, failures in cortical control of fronto-striatal neural circuits may underpin both compulsivity (OFC—dorsal striatum/caudate) and motor impulsivity (RIFC—globus pallidus), as well as reward-based impulsivity (ACC/VMPC—ventral striatum/NA shell), and contribute to these disorders. ACC, anterior cingulate cortex; NA, nucleus accumbens; OFC, orbitofrontal cortex; RIFC, right inferior frontal cortex; VLPFC, ventrolateral prefrontal cortex; VMPFC, ventromedial prefrontal cortex.

Accumulating evidence suggests that normal instrumental behaviour is governed by a balance between goal-directed (purposeful) actions and habitual actions (behaviours that are insensitive to the outcome value or environmental contingency change). After multiple repetitions, the habitual system renders purposeful behaviour automatic, allowing simple acts to be conducted without much effort. Goal-directed behaviour is mediated by the medial prefrontal/OFC and dorsal striatum (anterior caudate), whereas habitual actions involve the posterior lateral putamen. Evidence of an imbalance between these CSTC systems, coupled with an inappropriate shift from goal-directed action to habit in patients with OCD, suggests that altered habit learning may additionally contribute toward compulsive behaviours and introduces new possibilities for research and treatment (Gillan et al. 2014).

## 3.4 Neurochemistry

A range of evidence points to the role of the serotonin (5-HT) system in mediating OCD. The earliest evidence for this came from reports that clomipramine, a tricyclic antidepressant that is predominantly a 5-HT reuptake inhibitor (SRI), was effective in the treatment of OCD (Fernandez-Cordoba and Lopez-Ibor Alino 1967). These early reports were subsequently confirmed by controlled trials comparing clomipramine with noradrenergic reuptake inhibitors (Zohar and Insel 1987) and with placebo (DeVeaugh-Geiss et al. 1991). Clomipramine administration was shown to be accompanied by a decrease in cerebrospinal fluid (CSF) concentrations of the 5-HT metabolite 5-hydroxy-indoleacetic acid (CSF 5-HIAA) in OCD patients (Thoren et al. 1980).

Studies of static measures of serotonergic function in OCD have, however, been somewhat inconsistent, and other work has focused on more informative dynamic measures (Baumgarten and Grozdanovic 1998). Thus, for example, administration of the 5-HT agonist $m$-chloro-phenylpiperazine (mCPP) has been accompanied by exacerbation of OCD symptoms and a blunted neuroendocrine response in some (although not all) studies. Notably, after treatment with an SRI, behavioural and neuroendocrine responses to mCPP appear normalized (Zohar et al. 1988).

An immediate question is the possible role of specific 5-HT sub-receptors in OCD. Effects of mCPP on the post-synaptic 5-HT$_{2C}$ receptor, for example, may be particularly relevant to understanding its action in OCD (Bergqvist et al. 1999; Delgado and Moreno 1998). Preclinical data also suggest that the 5-HT$_{1D}$ terminal autoreceptor plays an important role; its desensitization in the OFC requires high duration/dose administration of SRIs, reminiscent of clinical findings (El Mansari et al. 1995). Preliminary challenge (Koran et al. 2001), pharmacological (Stern et al. 1998), genetic (Mundo et al. 2000), and imaging (Stein 1999) data support a role for 5-HT$_{1D}$ in OCD.

Molecular imaging, using ligand positron emission tomography (PET), offers an opportunity to visualize specific monoamine receptor occupancy in vivo. Molecular imaging studies of the 5-HT system in OCD are at an early stage, but further progress can be expected, as more serotonergic radioligands become available (Adams et al. 2005; Simpson et al. 2003). A systematic review of the relatively few PET ligand studies so far performed in OCD shows the strongest PET evidence supporting the involvement of the striatal post-synaptic dopamine D$_2$ receptor and the 5-HT transporter (SERT), with only inconsistent evidence of changes in 5-HT receptor binding potential. Studies in OCD focusing on SERT show decreased binding in cortical and subcortical areas (Hesse et al. 2011; Matsumoto et al. 2010; Reimold et al. 2007), related to a SERT polymorphism. Studies on the post-synaptic dopamine D$_2$ receptor in OCD, using [11C]-raclopride PET, showed decreased binding in the striatum in OCD (Moresco et al. 2007; Perani et al. 2008), normalizing (increasing) after treatment with an SSRI (Moresco et al. 2007).

Perhaps the most convincing evidence that serotonergic abnormalities can lead to OCD comes from genetic studies showing that, in a small percentage of OCD subjects, specific functional gene variants in the 5-HT system are associated with OCD (Ozaki et al. 2003). Recently, the combination of gene variants and imaging techniques has been explored as a tool for the enhancement of imaging findings. Several gene variants have been associated with structural and functional alteration in CSTC circuits relevant to OCRDs. For example, genetic variation in SERT was demonstrated to be associated in OCD with: (a) reduced OFC volume, as measured by magnetic resonance imaging (MRI) (Atmaca et al. 2011; Hesse et al. 2011), and (b) the availability of SERT in the putamen, nucleus accumbens, and hypothalamus, as measured by [11C]-DASB PET) (Hesse et al. 2011).

As above, another CSTC neurotransmitter system that may be particularly important in mediating OCD in some patients is dopamine (Goodman et al. 1990). In preclinical studies, administration of dopamine agonists leads to stereotypic behaviour, while, in humans, such agents may exacerbate OCD symptoms and tics (Denys et al. 2006). As noted, molecular imaging studies have documented altered binding in specific dopamine receptors in OCD (Denys et al. 2004; van der Wee et al. 2004). Conversely, dopamine blockers are used in the treatment of Tourette's syndrome, a putative OCD spectrum disorder. Furthermore, there is growing evidence that augmentation of SRIs with such agents may be useful in treatment-refractory OCD (Fineberg et al. 2013; Ipser et al. 2006). A recent study of deep brain stimulation in OCD, targeted at the nucleus accumbens, induced striatal dopamine release, which was associated with improved clinical symptoms, suggesting that CSTC stimulation compensates for a defective dopaminergic system (Figee et al. 2013).

Evidence is also accruing to support a role for glutamate transmission in the pathogenesis of OCD (Kariuki-Nyuthe et al. 2014). Glutamate is prominently represented in the CSTC circuitry (Bronstein and Cummings 2001). Results from MRS studies suggest the existence of an inverse relationship between glutamate levels in the anterior cingulate and striatum in symptomatic OCD, as well as a significant difference between pre-/post-treatment levels of glutamate in the caudate nucleus (Rosenberg et al. 2000). Treatments acting as partial agonists/antagonists at glutamate receptors, such as memantine and ketamine, may have a therapeutic role in OCD (reviewed in Fineberg et al. 2013; Grados et al. 2013).

A range of other transmitter systems, including certain neuropeptides (McDougle et al. 1999) and gonadal steroids (Alonso et al. 2011; Lochner and Stein 2001; Williams and Koran 1997) may, however, also play a role in OCD and related disorders. Ultimately, the role of second and third messenger pathways in these conditions will need to be fully delineated (Harvey et al. 2002; Marazziti et al. 2000; Perez et al. 2000).

## 3.5 Neurogenetics

Early work suggesting that OCD has a familial component has been confirmed by more recent rigorous studies that have used structured diagnostic interviews of probands and controls (Hettema et al. 2001; van Grootheest et al. 2005). Moreover, specific OCD symptom dimensions may share a familial relationship (Hasler et al. 2006, 2007) Also, several studies have demonstrated a genetic relationship between OCD and Tourette's syndrome (Pauls and Alsobrook 1999). Patients with OCD symptoms and a family history of Tourette's may have neurobiological dysfunction more similar to Tourette's than to primary OCD (Moriarty et al. 1997). Results from genome-wide studies indicate, however, that, while there is some genetic overlap between these two phenotypically related neuropsychiatric disorders, OCD and Tourette's have distinct genetic architectures (Davis et al. 2013). It is also worth noting that the only twin study, to date, in trichotillomania supported a role for genetic factors (Novak et al. 2009). Genetic findings in OCD spectrum disorders may ultimately lead to an understanding of a range of related conditions (Abelson et al. 2005; Zuchner et al. 2006). Patients with obsessive-compulsive symptoms secondary to chromosomal deletions may provide intriguing clues about which genes are involved in mediating the disorder (Gothelf et al. 2004).

Although there is increasing interest in the possibility that functional genetic polymorphisms may play a role in the pathogenesis of OCD (Hemmings and Stein 2006; Pato et al. 2001), the identification of causal gene variants has remained difficult (Walitza et al. 2010). As OCD has a complex aetiology, it is likely that multiple genes confer risk, each with small effect size. Although not all studies are consistent, there is accumulating evidence that polymorphisms in genes, including those involved in serotonergic (e.g. SERT), dopaminergic (e.g. catechol-O-methyltransferase) (Hemmings et al. 2004; Nicolini et al. 1998), and glutamatergic systems (e.g. SLC1A1), as well as other systems (e.g. opioid receptors, gamma aminobutyric acid (GABA) receptors, neurotrophic pathways, cell adhesion, and synaptic plasticity) (Table 3.2), may all contribute to vulnerability to OCD (Azzam and Mathews 2003; Hasler et al. 2006; Hemmings et al. 2002). In a recent meta-analysis, some risk genes were confirmed to be significantly associated with OCD (Taylor 2013).These include 5-HT-related polymorphisms (5-HTTLPR and HTR2A) and those related to catecholamine modulation (catechol-O-methyltransferase, COMT, and monoamine oxidase A, (MAOA)).Whole genome scanning has suggested that a number of chromosomal regions may be particularly important in OCD (Shugart et al. 2006) and has pointed to a number of new candidate genes (Stewart et al. 2013).

Recently, the combination of gene variants and imaging techniques has been explored as a tool for the enhancement of imaging findings. As noted earlier, several gene variants have been associated with structural and functional brain alteration relevant to OCRDs. For example, genetic variation in the SERT was demonstrated to be associated in OCD with: (a) reduced OFC volume, as measured by MRI (Atmaca et al. 2011; Hesse et al. 2011), and (b) the availability of the SERT in the putamen, nucleus accumbens, and hypothalamus, as measured by [11C]-DASB PET (Hesse et al. 2011).

A number of other approaches to determining the genetic basis of OCD may also yield important results. Animal models may be useful in suggesting a role for particular genes in stereotypic behaviour (Berridge et al. 2005). Earlier models show behavioural similarity to OCD and related compulsive behavioural disorders (for reviews, see d'Angelo et al. 2013; Fineberg et al. 2011) (Table 3.3). For instance, Hoxb8 mutant mice show excessive grooming behaviour that resembles trichotillomania. Dopamine transporter knock-down mice display excessively stereotyped and predictable grooming sequences, termed 'sequential super stereotypy', that superficially resemble the overly rigid sequential patterns of action, language, or thought displayed by patients with OCD and Tourette's syndrome. $5\text{-HT}_{2C}$ knockout mice also exhibit a range of compulsive-like behaviours, including increased chewing. While most of these models show some relevance (construct validity) to OCD, e.g. by demonstrating involvement of CSTC circuits, few have also demonstrated pharmacological predictive validity (Table 3.3).

In newer animal models, genetic alteration in regional glutamate signalling induces compulsive-like behaviours with pharmacological responses redolent of human OCD. These models offer better construct and predictive validity. In the mouse, SAP90/PSD95-associated protein 3 (Sapap3) is a post-synaptic scaffolding protein that is highly expressed in glutamatergic synapses of the striatum, a region implicated across obsessive-compulsive spectrum disorders. Sapap3 knockout mice show obsessive-compulsive-like behaviours, including excessive self-grooming and increased anxiety-like behaviours, which are additionally alleviated by repeated (6 days), but not acute, treatment with an SSRI. Loss of the neuron-specific transmembrane protein SLIT and NTRK-like protein-5 (Slitrk5) also leads to obsessive-compulsive-like behaviours in mice, including excessive self-grooming, increased anxiety-like behaviours, and increased marble burying, which was alleviated by chronic fluoxetine administration, supporting the relevance of this behaviour to OCD. The aromatase knockout (ArKO) mouse lacks a functioning aromatase enzyme and is therefore oestrogen-deficient. Male, but not female,

## Table 3.2 Population-/family-based association studies of candidate genes in OCD

| Candidate gene | Study design | Sample size | | | Significance |
| --- | --- | --- | --- | --- | --- |
| | | Cases | Controls | Families | |
| Dopamine receptor 4 | CC | 12 | 49 | – | P = 0.018 |
| | CC | 118 | 118 | – | P = 0.021 |
| | CC | 75 | 172 | – | P = 0.04 |
| | CC/FB | 49 | 63 | 34 | P = 0.03 |
| | CC | 71 | 129 | – | ns |
| | CC | 93 | 85 | – | P = 0.013 |
| Dopamine receptor 2 | CC | 67 | 54 | – | ns |
| | CC | 110 | 110 | – | P = 0.014 |
| Dopamine receptor 3 | CC | 97 | 97 | – | ns |
| | CC | 67 | 54 | – | ns |
| | CC | 103 | 103 | – | ns |
| Dopamine transporter | CC | 103 | 103 | – | ns |
| | CC | 75 | 172 | – | ns |
| | CC | 71 | 129 | – | ns |
| Monoamine oxidase A | FB | – | – | 110 | ns |
| | CC/FB | 122 | 124 | 51 | CC: P = 0.024 FB : P = 0.022 |
| | CC | 71 | 129 | – | ns |
| Catechol-O-methyltransferase | CC | 73 | 148 | – | P = 0.0002 |
| | FB | – | – | 10 | P = 0.0079 |
| | FB | – | – | 67 | P = 0.006 |
| | CC | 54 | 54 | – | P = 0.0017 |
| | FB | – | – | 56 | P = 0.048 |
| | CC | 17 | 35 | – | ns |
| | CC | 59 | 114 | – | ns |
| | CC | 144 | 337 | – | ns |
| | CC | 79 | 202 | – | ns |
| | CC | 373 | 462 | – | ns |
| Glutamate receptor subtype 2B | FB | – | – | 130 | P = 0.002 |
| Kainite glutamate receptor 2 | CC/FB | 156 | 156 | 141 | CC: ns FB: P = 0.03 |
| Gamma aminobutyric acid type B receptor 1 | FB | – | – | 159 | P = 0.006 |

(*continued*)

## Table 3.2 Continued

| Candidate gene | Study design | Sample size | | | Significance |
|---|---|---|---|---|---|
| | | Cases | Controls | Families | |
| Brain-derived neuro-trophic factor | FB | – | – | 164 | P <0.020 |
| | FB | – | – | 54 | ns |
| | CC | 347 | 749 | – | ns |
| Myelin oligodendrocyte | FB | – | – | 160 | P = 0.022 |
| Glutamate transporter | FB | – | – | 157 | P = 0.006 |
| | FB | – | – | 71 | P = 0.030 |
| | FB | – | – | 66 | P = 0.0015 |
| | CC | 325 | 662 | – | P <0.001 |
| | CC | 378 | 281 | – | ns |
| Oligodendrocyte lineage transcription factor 2 | FB | – | – | 66 | P = 0.004 |
| Neurotrophin-3 receptor gene (NTRK3) | CC | 153 | 324 | – | P = 0.005 |
| Extraneuronal mono-amine transporter, EMT (SLC22A3) | CC | 84 | 204 | | ns |
| SAPAP3 | CC | 172 | 153 | | P = 0.036 |
| Serotonin transporter | FB | – | – | 35 | P <0.03 |
| | CC | 75 | 397 | – | P = 0.023 |
| | CC | 75 | 172 | – | ns |
| | CC | 54 | 82 | – | ns |
| | CC | 156 | 134 | – | ns |
| | FB | – | – | 54 | ns |
| | CC | 99 | 420 | – | ns |
| | CC | 347 | 749 | – | ns |
| | CC | 295 | 657 | – | P <0.018 |
| Serotonin transporter promoter | CC | 129 | 479 | – | ns |
| | CC/FB | 115 | 136 | 43 | ns |
| | CC | 180 | 112 | – | ns |
| | FB | – | – | 63 | ns |
| | CC | 79 | 202 | – | ns |
| | CC/FB | 106 | 171 | 86 | ns |

(continued)

## Table 3.2 Continued

| Candidate gene | Study design | Sample size | | | Significance |
|---|---|---|---|---|---|
| | | Cases | Controls | Families | |
| Serotonin receptor 2A | CC | 67 | 54 | – | ns |
| | CC | 62 | 144 | – | P <0.05 |
| | CC | 101 | 138 | – | P = 0.015 |
| | CC | 75 | 172 | – | ns |
| | CC | 55 | 123 | – | ns |
| | CC | 71 | 129 | – | ns |
| | CC | ? | ? | – | ns |
| | CC | 58 | 83 | – | ns |
| | CC | 79 | 202 | – | P <0.00007 |
| | CC | 156 | 134 | – | ns |
| | FB | – | – | 54 | ns |
| | CC | 99 | 420 | – | P = 0.02 |
| Serotonin receptor 2C | CC | 109 | 107 | – | ns |
| | CC | 75 | 172 | – | ns |
| | CC | 79 | 202 | – | ns |
| Serotonin receptor 1B | FB | – | – | 32 | P <0.006 |
| | FB | – | – | 121 | P = 0.023 |
| | FB | – | – | 48 | ns |
| | CC | 77 | 129 | – | ns |
| | FB | – | – | 47 | ns |
| | FB | – | – | 63 | ns |
| | CC | 156 | 134 | – | ns |
| | FB | – | – | 54 | ns |

CC, population-based (case-control); FB, family-based; ns, non-significant finding; P, p value.

(Reproduced from *Obsessive-Compulsive Disorder: Current Science and Clinical Practice*, Edited by Joseph Zohar, Copyright (2012), with permission from John Wiley and Sons.)

ArKO mice develop compulsive behaviours, such as excessive barbering, grooming, and wheel running, all of which were normalized by 17beta-estradiol. This was paralleled by a significant decrease in COMT protein expression in the hypothalamus in male knockouts. COMT is one of the major enzymes involved in the metabolic degradation of catecholamines across species. The aromatase model describes a possible link between oestrogen, COMT, and the development of compulsive behaviours in male animals, which may have therapeutic implications in OCD patients.

Optogenetics is a neuromodulation strategy that combines techniques from optics and genetics. Targeted optical radiation is used to control and monitor the activities of individual neurons in freely moving animals and may be applied as a basis for experimental manipulation

| Table 3.3 Animal models in obsessive-compulsive spectrum disorders | | | | |
|---|---|---|---|---|
| Animal models | Description | Face validity | Construct validity (neurotransmitter/ anatomical abnormalities of OCD* and OCRD**) | Predictive validity |
| Genetic model | Hox B8 knockout mice: excessive auto-grooming | ++ TTM*** + (OCD) | + (gene expression in brain areas implicated in OCD) | ? |
| | Slitrk5 knockout mice: excessive auto-grooming, anxious behaviour | ++ (TTM) ++ (OCD) | ++ (increased FosB expression in orbito-frontal cortex (OFC); anatomical abnormalities in striatum) | + response to fluoxetine |
| | Sapap3 knockout mice: excessive auto-grooming, anxious behaviour | ++ (TTM) ++ (OCD) | ++ (involvement in OCD, expressed in glutamate systems) | + response to fluoxetine |
| | Serotonin 2c receptor knockout mice: compulsive behaviours | +/− (OCD) | + (5-HT$_{2c}$ receptor involvement in OCD; 5-HT abnormalities) | ? |
| | Dopamine transporter knock-down mice: elevated dopamine levels | +/− (OCD), (TS)**** | ++ (elevated free dopamine levels; striatal dopamine involvement in OCD, TTM) | ? |
| | D1CT mice: transgenic mice expressing cholera toxin—repetitive biting and leaping behaviour | + (OCD, TS) | + (transgene expressed in regions implicated in OCD) | ? |
| | Aromatase knockout mice: oestrogen-deficient: excessive barbering, grooming, and wheel-running | + (TTM) +/− (OCD) | + (associated with low COMT***** activity; evidence for involvement of oestradiol in OCD) | ? |
| Pharmacological models | Chronic quinpirole leads to excessive checking | ++ (OCD) | ++ (dopamine/5-HT involvement in OCD) + (reduced by high-frequency stimulation (HFS) of subthalamic nucleus, nucleus accumbens) − (no change with OFC lesions) | + (response to clomipramine) |
| | Acute 8-hydroxy-2-(di-ni-polylamino)-tetraline hydrobromide (8-OHDPAT) leads to perseveration | +/− (OCD) and motor perseveration relevant to other disorders | + (5-HT$_{1a}$ involvement in OCD) − (no change with HFS of thalamic reticular nucleus or OFC lesions) | + (response to fluoxetine) |

| | | | | |
|---|---|---|---|---|
| | Meta-chlorophenylpiperazine (mCPP)-induced directional persistence | +/− (OCD) and motor perseveration relevant to other disorders | + (5-HT involvement; 5-HT$_{2c}$ receptor involvement in OCD) | ++ (response to fluoxetine, but not to desipramine or diazepam) |
| | Clomipramine administration in neonatal rats leads to compulsive behaviours in later life | ++ (OCD) | ++ (increased 5-HT$_{2c}$ mRNA expression in the OFC; increased D2 mRNA expression in the striatum) | ? |
| | 5-HT$_{1b}$ agonist-induced compulsive-like behaviour | + (OCD) | ++ (involvement of OFC, 5-HT$_{1b}$ receptor involvement in OCD; 5-HT involvement) | ++ (response to fluoxetine and clomipramine) |
| | Quinpirole-induced excessive lever-pressing in rats | ++ (OCD) | + (involvement of dopamine) | ++ (response to clomipramine) |
| Behavioural models (ethological) | Acral lick dermatitis, hair-pulling in cats, feather-picking in birds following sensory deprivation/neglect | ++ (TTM) | ++ (spontaneous development) | Selective to fluoxetine/clomipramine, but not to desipramine |
| | Dogs with compulsive behaviours (tail-chasing, biting, and circling) | + (OCD) | + (involvement of striatum, frontal cortex, thalamus) ++ (involvement of 5-HT, dopamine) | +++ (response to fluoxetine, clomipramine, and memantine) |
| | Barbering in mice | +++ (TTM) | ++ (spontaneous development) | ? |
| | Spontaneous stereotypies in deer mice | +/− OCD, stereotypy in other disorders | ++ (spontaneous development) | ++ (response to fluoxetine, but not to desipramine) |
| Behavioural models (experimental) | Marble-burying in mice and rats | +/− (OCD; marble-burying cannot differentiate between anti-compulsive and anxiolytic activity) | ++ (modulation by sex steroids; involvement of 5-HT, dopamine; involvement of NMDA receptors, nitric oxide) | +++ (response to SSRIs, memantine, and aripiprazole, but not to desipramine) |
| | Attenuation of a feedback cue-signalling reward delivery leads to excessive lever-pressing, not followed by attempts to collect the reward | ++ (OCD) | + (deficient psychological process implicated in OCD) ++ (involvement of OFC, striatum) ++ (involvement of 5-HT, dopamine, glutamate; modulation by sex steroids) | +++ (response to fluoxetine and-cycloserine, but not to desipramine) |

(continued)

| Table 3.3 Continued | | | | |
|---|---|---|---|---|
| Animal models | Description | Face validity | Construct validity (neurotransmitter/anatomical abnormalities of OCD* and OCRD**) | Predictive validity |
| | Perseveration in reversal learning | +/– (OCD: motor perseveration relevant to other disorders as well) | + (OFC lesions increase perseveration)<br>++ (OCD-associated candidate endophenotype)<br>+++ (5-HT involvement) | + (response to citalopram)<br>– (response to atomoxetine and desipramine) |
| | Impaired shifting of attentional focus between stimulus dimensions | ++ (OCD) | ++ (OCD-associated candidate endophenotype)<br>+ (brain areas implicated in OCD)<br>– (no involvement of 5-HT)<br>– (noradrenaline abnormality) | + (response to escitalopram, quetiapine)<br>– (response to desipramine) |
| | Impaired suppression of pre-potent motor responses | ++ (OCD, TTM) | + (deficient psychological process implicated in OC spectrum)<br>++ (OCD-associated candidate endophenotype)<br>+ (brain areas implicated in OCD, TTM)<br>– (no involvement of 5-HT; involvement of noradrenaline) | – (response to atomoxetine)<br>No response to citalopram |

* Obsessive-compulsive disorder.

** Obsessive-compulsive related disorders.

*** Tourette's syndrome.

**** Catechol-o-methyl transferase.

? Not known.

(Reproduced from CNS Spectr., **19**(1), Camilla d'Angelo LS, Eagle DM, Grant JE, et al., Animal models of obsessive-compulsive spectrum disorders, p. 28–49, Copyright (2013), with permission from Cambridge University Press.)

of cortico-striatal function. In one recent study, repetitive (but not acute) optogenetic orbitofrontal cortex (OFC)–ventromedial striatum (VMS) stimulation in mice generated a progressive increase in grooming, which persisted for 2 weeks after stimulation cessation. The grooming increase was temporally coupled with a progressive increase in light-evoked firing of post-synaptic VMS cells. Both increased grooming and evoked firing were reversed by chronic fluoxetine administration, a first-line OCD treatment (Ahmari et al. 2013). In another study, focused optogenetic stimulation of the lateral OFC and its terminals in the striatum restored abnormal behavioural response inhibition and defective downregulation, and compensated for impaired fast-spiking neuron striatal microcircuits in a Sapap3 mouse model of compulsive grooming behaviour (Burguière et al. 2013). These findings further implicate abnormal CSTC activity in the generation of sustained compulsive psychopathology and suggest potential for the design of targeted treatments for compulsive disorders.

## 3.6 Neuroimmunology

Early reports of an association between OCD and Sydenham's chorea were confirmed in a systematic investigation (Swedo et al. 1989), leading to a consideration of whether some cases of OCD involve autoimmune processes that disrupt CSTC circuits. It is specifically proposed that antibodies raised against streptococcal proteins cross-react with neuronal proteins (antigens) in the brain, particularly in the basal ganglia (Swedo et al. 1998). Indeed, the term 'paediatric autoimmune neuropsychiatric disorder associated with streptococcal infections' (PANDAS) has been coined to describe patients who have acute onset of OCD symptoms and/or tics in the aftermath of streptococcal infection (Swedo et al. 1998).

This seminal contribution was followed by a series of studies exploring various aspects of an autoimmune hypothesis of OCD (Leonard and Swedo 2001). Patients with suspected PANDAS, for example, were shown to demonstrate abnormal striatal volume on brain imaging (Giedd et al. 2000). Furthermore, their OCD and tic symptoms responded to immunomodulatory interventions such as plasma exchange and intravenous immunoglobulin. Long-term follow-up revealed continued symptom improvement for the majority of patients, particularly when antibiotic prophylaxis had been effective in preventing recurrent streptococcal infections (Snider et al. 2005).

However, despite two decades of research, uncertainties about the clinical definition of PANDAS remain, and the available evidence does not convincingly support the disorder as a well-defined clinical entity. Moreover, there is still rather limited evidence supporting the efficacy of antibiotic or immunoglobulin treatment in those with PANDAS. Larger prospective studies are required to elucidate the exact nature of disease mechanisms of post-streptococcal neuropsychiatric disorders other than Sydenham's chorea (Singer et al. 2012; Swedo et al. 2012).

Nevertheless, there is evidence of a number of immune dysfunctions in OCD, including abnormal auto-antibodies in some (but not all) studies (Stein et al. 2000). One such study found increased levels of anti-basal ganglia antibodies in approximately 20% of adult patients with OCD (compared with 4% of psychiatric controls; Fisher's exact test $P = 0.012$), but there was no evidence to link this with streptococcal infection (Nicholson et al. 2012). These findings support the hypothesis that central nervous system autoimmunity may have an aetiological role in some adults with OCD. However, the putative association between immune dysfunctions and OCD requires further study to determine its specificity (versus other disorders) (Harel et al. 2001), its frequency (compared with other possible striatal insults), and its relationship to other psychobiological factors (such as genetic variables) (Lougee et al. 2000). To this end, work on the autoimmune hypothesis of OCD is ongoing, with the aim of establishing the precise immunological mechanisms involved (Swedo and Grant 2005). Expression of D8/17, a B-lymphocyte antigen and marker of susceptibility to developing sequelae after streptococcal infection, was found to be increased in some (but not all) studies of OCD (Brimberg et al. 2012; Eisen et al. 2001; Merlo et al. 2005; Nicholson et al. 2012). In addition, specific polymorphisms of the promoter region of tumour necrosis factor (TNF)-alpha gene have been associated with OCD occurring after rheumatic fever (Sampaio et al. 2013).

Altogether, work in this area has strengthened the current view of OCD as a neuropsychiatric disorder and may ultimately lead to the identification of at-risk children and novel treatments.

## 3.7 Neuroethology

A range of work has been done to develop animal models of the proximal neurobiological mechanisms relevant to understanding habits (Graybiel and Rauch 2000) and OCD (D'angelo et al. 2013; Joel 2006) (Table 3.3). There is also interest in the idea that an evolutionary perspective may provide an understanding of the distal survival mechanisms that are relevant to the disorder. A number of authors have noted that OCD symptoms are redolent of animal stereotypies, that the striatum is a repository for patterned motoric sequences, and that there is an overlap in the neurochemistry mediating stereotypies and OCD (Berridge et al. 2005; Ridley 1994).

A particularly intriguing set of ethological animal models is that found in veterinary behavioural practice (Dodman et al. 1997). Acral lick dermatitis in dogs, for example, is characterized by repetitive licking of the paws that is reminiscent of some cases of OCD, in which the hands are licked, rather than washed. The condition appears commoner in certain canine families, and its pharmacotherapy response profile is remarkably similar to that of OCD (Rapoport et al. 1992). Other models of OCD and spectrum disorders include barbering in mice, feather picking in birds, and cribbing in horses (Garner et al. 2003, 2004).

Other findings from the animal literature suggest a role for environmental factors in promoting stereotypies (Ridley 1994). Stereotypic behaviour can, for example, be induced by confinement or by emotional deprivation. Interestingly, primates raised under conditions of deprivation demonstrate abnormalities in striatal architecture (Martin et al. 1991). The SSRI fluoxetine is more effective than placebo in the pharmacotherapy of stereotypies in deprived non-human primates (Hugo et al. 2003).

Indeed, an ethological perspective has generated a range of hypotheses about OCD (Leckman and Mayes 1999). Although speculative, these are arguably valuable insofar as they help supplement work on the proximate mechanisms of OCD with ideas about its ultimate evolutionary underpinnings. One thought-provoking set of research has focused on disgust (Stein et al. 2001); fear and disgust are mediated by different pathways—while the amygdala is crucial in mediating fear in a number of anxiety disorders (Cannistratio et al. 2004), CSTC and other circuits may be responsible for impairments in disgust processing in OCD. Imaging studies of disgust processing in OCD patients are consistent with the idea that disruption in this key emotion is important in OCD (Shapira et al. 2003).

## 3.8 Integration

This chapter has summarized a broad range of evidence which emphasizes the role of CSTC circuits in mediating OCD. Further work is, however, ongoing to establish the exact origins and nature of CSTC dysfunction; such research incorporates various kinds of data, including neuroanatomic, neurocognitive, neurochemical, neurogenetic, neuroimmunological, and neuroethological variables. In the interim, attempts can be made to integrate what is known about the role of CSTC circuits in general neuropsychological processing with an understanding of OCD and related disorders.

An early neuroanatomical hypothesis, for example, was that caudate abnormalities were associated with cognitive symptoms (such as are apparent in OCD), whereas putamen dysfunction led to sensorimotor symptoms (such as the tics of Tourette's syndrome) (Rauch and Baxter 1998). However, imaging research suggests that a wider range of different CSTC circuits are involved in OCD (Rosenberg and Keshavan 1998), including systems responsible for reward processing more usually associated with addiction (Klanker et al. 2013). Possibly, specific projection fields or cell types may be involved in particular kinds of behavioural phenomena and clinical symptoms (Barnes et al. 2005). Certainly, CSTC circuits play a role in mediating the development, maintenance, and selection of procedural strategies (Graybiel 1998; Saint-Cyr et al. 1995). CSTC circuits appear to play a particularly important role in recognizing behaviourally significant stimuli (and in error detection) and in regulating goal-directed responses (including response inhibition and habit learning) (Davidson et al. 2001; Lovinger 2010; Rauch and Baxter 1998; Zald and Kim 1996), and may therefore be particularly important in OCD.

It has been suggested that OCD involves a failure to inhibit CSTC-mediated procedural strategies from intruding into consciousness (Stein 2002). Such a view appears consistent with: (1) the limited number of symptom themes in OCD, and their apparent evolutionary importance; (2) the dysfunction of CSTC circuits in OCD, with activation of temporal, rather than striatal, areas during implicit cognition (Rauch et al. 2001); (3) the role of the 5-HT in particular and interrelated neurotransmitter systems in general, as the 5-HT system in CSTC circuits is thought to play an important role in mediating inhibitory processes; (4) evidence of disinhibitory and habitual processes in OCD and related conditions (Chamberlain et al. 2005; Fineberg et al. 2014). Much further research is nevertheless needed to fully delineate the cognitive–affective neuroscience of OCD and related disorders.

# References

Abelson JF, et al. (2005). Sequence variants in SLITRK1 are associated with Tourette's syndrome. *Science.* **310**: 317–20.

Adams KH, et al. (2005). Patients with obsessive–compulsive disorder have increased 5-HT2A receptor binding in the caudate nuclei. *Int J Neuropsychopharmacol.* **8**: 391–401.

Ahmari SE, et al. (2013). Repeated cortico-striatal stimulation generates persistent OCD-like behavior. *Science.* **340**: 1234–9.

Alonso P, et al. (2011). Variants in estrogen receptor alpha gene are associated with phenotypical expression of obsessive–compulsive disorder. *Psychoneuroendocrinology.* **36**: 473–83.

Arnold PD, et al. (2004). Association of a glutamate (NMDA) subunit receptor gene (GRIN2B) with obsessive–compulsive disorder: a preliminary study. *Psychopharmacologia.* **174**: 530–8.

Arnold PD, et al. (2006). Glutamate transporter gene SLC1A1 associated with obsessive–compulsive disorder. *Arch Gen Psychiatry.* **63**: 769–76.

Atmaca M, et al. (2011). Serotonin transporter gene polymorphism implicates reduced orbito-frontal cortex in obsessive–compulsive disorder. *J Anxiety Disord.* **25**: 680–5.

Azzam A and Mathews CA (2003). Meta-analysis of the association between the catecholamine-O-methyl-transferase gene and obsessive–compulsive disorder. *Am J Med Genet B Neuropsychiat Genet.* **123**: 64–9.

Barnes TD, et al. (2005). Activity of striatal neurons reflects dynamic encoding and recoding of procedural memories. *Nature.* **437**: 1158–61.

Baumgarten HG and Grozdanovic Z (1998). Role of serotonin in obsessive–compulsive disorder. *Br J Psychiat.ry.* **Suppl. 35**, 13–20.

Baxter LR, et al. (1992). Caudate glucose metabolic rate changes with both drug and behavior therapy for OCD. Arch Gen Psychiat. **49**: 681–9.

Benazon NR, Moore GJ, and Rosenberg DR (2003). Neurochemical analyses in pediatric obsessive–compulsive disorder in patients treated with cognitive-behavioral therapy. J Am Acad Child Adolesc Psychiatry. **42**: 1279–85.

Bergqvist PB, et al. (1999). Effect of atypical antipsychotic drugs on 5-HT2 receptors in the rat orbito-frontal cortex: an in vivo electrophysiological study. Psychopharmacology. **143**: 89–96.

Berridge KC, et al. (2005). Sequential super-stereotypy of an instinctive fixed action pattern in hyper-dopaminergic mutant mice: a model of obsessive compulsive disorder and Tourette's. BMC Biol. **3**: 4.

Bourne SK, et al. (2012). Mechanisms of deep brain stimulation in for obsessive compulsive disorder: effects upon cells and circuits. Front Integr Neurosci. **6**: 29.

Brewer JA and Potenza MN (2008). The neurobiology and genetics of impulse control disorders: relationships to drug addictions. Biochem Pharmacol. **75**: 63–75.

Brimberg L, et al. (2012). Behavioral, pharmacological, and immunological abnormalities after streptococcal exposure: a novel rat model of Sydenham chorea and related neuropsychiatric disorders. Neuropsychopharmacol. **37**: 2076–87.

Brody AL, et al. (1998). FDG-PET predictors of response to behavioral therapy and pharmacotherapy in obsessive compulsive disorder. Psychiat Res. **84**: 1–6.

Bronstein Y and Cummings J (2001). Neurochemistry of frontal-subcortical circuits. In: Lichter D, Cummings J, eds. Frontal-Subcortical Circuits in Psychiatric and Neurological Disorders. New York: Guilford Press, pp. 59–91.

Burguière E, et al. (2013). Optogenetic stimulation of lateral orbito-fronto-striatal pathway suppresses compulsive behaviours. Science. **340**: 1243–6.

Cannistraro PA, et al. (2004). Amygdala responses to human faces in obsessive–compulsive disorder. Biol Psychiatry. **56**: 916–20.

Chamberlain SR and Menzies L (2009). Endophenotypes of obsessive–compulsive disorder: rationale, evidence and future potential. Expert Rev Neurother. **9**: 1133–46.

Chamberlain SR, et al. (2005). The neuropsychology of obsessive compulsive disorder: the importance of failures in cognitive and behavioural inhibition as candidate endophenotypic markers. Neurosci Biobehav Rev. **29**: 399–419.

Chamberlain SR, et al. (2008). Orbitofrontal dysfunction in patients with obsessive–compulsive disorder and their unaffected relatives. Science. **18**; 321: 421–2.

Cheyette SR and Cummings JL (1995). Encephalitis lethargica: lessons for contemporary neuropsychiatry. J Neuropsychiat Clin Neurosci. **7**: 125–35.

d'Angelo LS, et al. (2013). Animal models of obsessive–compulsive spectrum disorders. CNS Spectr. **19**: 28–49.

Davidson RJ, et al. (2001). Dysfunction in the neural circuitry of emotion regulation—a possible prelude to violence. Science. **289**: 591–4.

Davis LK, et al. (2013). Partitioning the heritability of Tourette syndrome and obsessive compulsive disorder reveals differences in genetic architecture. PLoS Genet. **9**: e1003864.

Delgado PL and Moreno FA (1998). Hallucinogens, serotonin and obsessive–compulsive disorder. J Psychoactive Drugs. **30**: 359–66.

Denys D, et al. (2004). The role of dopamine in obsessive–compulsive disorder: preclinical and clinical evidence. J Clin Psychiatry. **65**: 11–17.

Denys D, et al. (2013). Dopaminergic activity in Tourette syndrome and obsessive–compulsive disorder. Eur Neuropsychopharmacol. **23**: 1423–31.

DeVeaugh-Geiss J, et al. (1991). Clomipramine in the treatment of patients with obsessive–compulsive disorder: the clomipramine collaborative study group. Arch Gen Psychiatry. **48**: 730–8.

de Wit SJ, et al. (2014). Multicenter voxel-based morphometry mega-analysis of structural brain scans in obsessive–compulsive disorder. Am J Psychiatry. **171**: 340–9.

Dodman NH, et al. (1997). Animal models of obsessive–compulsive disorder. In: Hollander E, Stein DJ, eds. Obsessive–Compulsive Disorders: Diagnosis, Etiology, Treatment. New York: Marcel Dekker.

Eisen JL, et al. (2001). The use of antibody D8/17 to identify B cells in adults with obsessive–compulsive disorder. Psychiatry Res. **104**: 221–5.

El Mansari, *et al.* (1995). Alteration of serotonin release in the guinea pig orbito-frontal cortex by selective serotonin reuptake inhibitors. *Neuropsychopharmacol.* **13**: 117–27.

Fernandez-Cordoba E and Lopez-Ibor Alino J (1967). [La monoclorimipramina en enfermos psiquiatricos resistentes a otros tratamientos]. *Acta Luso-Esp Neurol Psiquiat Ciene Afines.* **26**: 119–47.

Figee M, *et al.* (2013). Deep brain stimulation restores frontostriatal network activity in obsessive–compulsive disorder. *Nature Neuroscience.* **16**: 386–7.

Fineberg NA, *et al.* (2010). Probing compulsive and impulsive behaviors, from animal models to endopheno-types: a narrative review. *Neuropsychopharmacol.* **35**: 591–604.

Fineberg N, *et al.* (2011). Translational approaches to obsessive–compulsive disorder: from animal models to clinical treatment. *Br J Pharmacol.* **164**: 1044–61.

Fineberg NA, *et al.* (2013). Pharmacotherapy of obsessive–compulsive disorder: evidence-based treatment and beyond. *Aust N Z J Psychiatry.* **47**:121–41.

Fineberg NA, *et al.* (2014). New developments in human neurocognition: impulsivity and compulsivity. *CNS Spectr.* **19**: 69–89.

Garner JP, *et al.* (2003). Stereotypies in caged parrots, schizophrenia and autism: evidence for a common mechanism. *Behav Brain Res.* **145**: 125–34.

Garner JP, *et al.* (2004). Barbering (fur and whisker trimming) by laboratory mice as a model of human trichotillomania and obsessive–compulsive spectrum disorders. *Comp Med.* **54**: 216–24.

Giedd JN, *et al.* (2000). MRI assessment of children with obsessive–compulsive disorder or tics associated with streptococcal infection. *Am J Psychiat.* **157**: 281–3.

Gillan CM, *et al.* (2014). Enhanced avoidance habits in obsessive–compulsive disorder. *Biol Psychiatry.* **75**: 631–8.

Goodman WK, *et al.* (1990). Beyond the serotonin hypothesis: a role for dopamine in some forms of obsessive–compulsive disorder. *J Clin Psychiatry.* **51S**: 36–43.

Gothelf D, *et al.* (2004). Obsessive–compulsive disorder in patients with velocardiofacial (22q11 deletion) syndrome. *Am J Med Genet.* **B126**: 99–105.

Grados MA, *et al.* (2013). Glutamate drugs and pharmacogenetics of OCD: a pathway-based exploratory approach. *Expert Opin Drug Discov.* **8**: 1515–27.

Graybiel AM (1998). The basal ganglia and chunking of action repertoires. *Neurobiol Learn Mem.* **70**: 119–36.

Graybiel AM and Rauch SL (2000). Toward a neurobiology of obsessive–compulsive disorder. *Neuron.* **28**: 343–7.

Harel Z, *et al.* (2001). Antibodies against human putamen in adolescents with anorexia nervosa. *Int J Eat Disord.* **29**: 463–9.

Harvey BH, *et al.* (2002). Defining the neuromolecular action of myoinositol: application to obsessive–compulsive disorder. *Prog Neuro-Psychopharmacol Biol Psychiatry.* **26**: 21–32.

Hasler G, *et al.* (2006). Factor analysis of obsessive–compulsive disorder YBOCS-SC symptoms and association with 5-HTTLPR SERT polymorphism. *Am J Med Genet.* **B141**: 403–8.

Hasler G, *et al.* (2007). OCD Collaborative Genetics Study. Familiality of factor analysis-derived YBOCS dimensions in OCD-affected sibling pairs from the OCD Collaborative Genetics Study. *Biol Psychiatry.* **61**: 617–25.

Hemmings SMJ and Stein DJ (2006). The current status of association studies in obsessive–compulsive disorder. *Psychiat Clin North Amer.* **29**: 411–44.

Hemmings SMJ, *et al.* (2002). Dopaminergic and serotonergic system genes in obsessive–compulsive disorder: a case-control association study in the Afrikaner population. Unpublished.

Hemmings SM, *et al.* (2004). Early- versus late-onset obsessive–compulsive disorder: investigating genetic and clinical correlates. *Psychiat Res.* **128**: 175–82.

Hesse S, *et al.* (2011). The serotonin transporter availability in untreated early-onset and late-onset patients with obsessive–compulsive disorder. *Int J Neuropsychopharmacol.* **14**: 606–17.

Hettema JM, *et al.* (2001). A review and meta-analysis of the genetic epidemiology of anxiety disorders. *Am J Psychiat.* **158**: 1568–78.

Hoexter MQ, *et al.* (2013). Differential prefrontal gray matter correlates of treatment response to fluoxetine or cognitive-behavioral therapy in obsessive–compulsive disorder. *Eur Neuropsychopharm.* **23**: 569–80.

Hollander E and Wong CM (1995). Obsessive–compulsive spectrum disorders. *J Clin Psychiatry.* **56**: 3–6.

Hugo F, et al. (1999). Functional brain imaging in obsessive–compulsive disorder secondary to neurological lesions. *Depress Anxiety*. **10**: 129–36.

Hugo C, et al. (2003). Fluoxetine decreases stereotypic behavior in primates. *Prog Neuropsychopharmacol Biol Psychiatry*. **27**: 639–43.

Ipser JC, et al. (2006). Pharmacotherapy augmentation strategies in treatment-resistant anxiety disorders. *Cochrane Database Syst Rev*. CD005473.

Jenike MA (1998). Neurosurgical treatment of obsessive–compulsive disorder. *Br J Psychiatry*. **Suppl.35**: 79–90.

Joel D (2006). Current animal models of obsessive–compulsive disorder: a critical review. *Prog Neuropsychopharmacol Biol Psychiat*. **30**: 374–88.

Kariuki-Nyuthe C, et al. (2014). Obsessive compulsive disorder and the glutamate system. *Curr Opin Psychiatry*. **27**: 32–7.

Klanker M, et al. (2013). Dopaminergic control of cognitive flexibility in humans and animals. *Front Neurosci*. **7**: 201.

Koran LM, et al. (2001). Sumatriptan, 5-HT (1D) receptors and obsessive–compulsive disorder. *Eur Neuropsychopharmacol*. **11**: 169–72.

Leckman JF and Mayes LC (1999). Preoccupations and behaviors associated with romantic and parental love. Perspectives on the origin of obsessive–compulsive disorder. *Child Adolesc Psychiat Clin North Amer*. **8**: 635–65.

Leonard HL and Swedo SE (2001). Paediatric autoimmune neuropsychiatric disorders associated with streptococcal infection (PANDAS). *Int J Neuropsychopharmacol*. **4**: 191–8.

Lochner C and Stein DJ (2001). Gender in obsessive–compulsive disorder and obsessive–compulsive spectrum disorders. *Archs Women's Mental Hlth*. **4**: 19–26.

Lougee L, et al. (2000). Psychiatric disorders in first-degree relatives of children with pediatric autoimmune neuropsychiatric disorders associated with streptococcal infections (PANDAS). *J Am Acad Child Adolesc Psychiat*. **39**: 1120–6.

Lovinger DM. (2010) Neurotransmitter roles in synaptic modulation, plasticity and learning in the dorsal striatum. *Neuropharmacology*. **58**: 951–61.

Marazziti D, et al. (2000). Increased inhibitory activity of protein kinase C on the serotonin transporter in OCD. *Neuropsychobiology*. **41**: 171–7.

Martin LJ, et al. (1991). Social deprivation of infant monkeys alters the chemoarchitecture of the brain: I. Subcortical regions. *J Neurosci*. **11**: 3344–58.

Mataix-Cols D, Rosario-Campos MC, and Leckman JF (2005). A multidimensional model of obsessive–compulsive disorder. *Am J Psychiatry*, **162**: 228–38.

Matsumoto R, et al. (2010). Reduced serotonin transporter binding in the insular cortex in patients with obsessive–compulsive disorder: A [11C]DASB PET study. *Neuroimage*. **49**: 121–6.

McDougle CJ, et al. (1999). Possible role of neuropeptides in obsessive compulsive disorder. *Psychoneuroendocrinology*. **24**: 1–24.

Menzies L, et al. (2007). Neurocognitive endophenotypes of obsessive–compulsive disorder. *Brain*. **130**: 3223–36.

Menzies L, et al. (2008). Integrating evidence from neuroimaging and neuropsychological studies of obsessive–compulsive disorder: the orbitofronto-striatal model revisited. *Neurosci Biobehav Rev*. **32**: 525 49.

Merlo LJ, et al. (2005). Assessment of pediatric obsessive–compulsive disorder: a critical review of current methodology. *Child Psychiat Hum Dev*. **36**: 195–214.

Meunier D, et al. (2012). Brain functional connectivity in stimulant drug dependence and obsessive–compulsive disorder. *Neuroimage*. **59**: 1461–8.

Morein-Zamir S, et al. (2010). Inhibition of thoughts and actions in obsessive–compulsive disorder: extending the endophenotype? *Psychol Med*. **40**: 263–72.

Moresco RM, et al. (2007). Fluvoxamine treatment and D2 receptors: a PET study on OCD drug-naïve patients. *Neuropsychopharmacol*. **32**: 197–205.

Moriarty J, et al. (1997). HMPAO SPET does not distinguish obsessive–compulsive and tic syndromes in families multiply affected with Gilles de la Tourette's syndrome. *Psychol Med*. **27**: 737–40.

Mundo E, et al. (2000). Is the 5-HT (1Dbeta) receptor gene implicated in the pathogenesis of obsessive–compulsive disorder? Am J Psychiatry. **157**: 1160–1.

Nicholson TR, et al. (2012). Prevalence of anti-basal ganglia antibodies in adult obsessive–compulsive disorder: cross-sectional study. Br J Psychiatry. **200**: 381–6.

Nicolini H, et al. (1998). Dopamine D2 and D4 receptor genes distinguish the clinical presence of tics in obsessive–compulsive disorder. Gac Med Mex. **134**: 521–7.

Novak CE, et al. (2009). A twin concordance study of trichotillomania. Am J Med Genet B Neuropsychiatr Genet. **50B**: 944–9.

Ozaki N, et al. (2003). Serotonin transporter missense mutation associated with a complex neuropsychiatric phenotype. Mol Psychiatry. **8**: 895, 933–6.

Pato MT, et al. (2001). The genetics of obsessive–compulsive disorder. Curr Psychiatry Rep. **3**: 163–8.

Pauls DL and Alsobrook JP 2nd (1999). The inheritance of obsessive–compulsive disorder. Child Adolesc Psychiatr Clin North Amer. **8**: 481–96.

Perani D, et al. (2008). In vivo PET study of 5HT2A serotonin and D2 dopamine dysfunction in drug-naive obsessive–compulsive disorder. Neuroimage. **42**: 306–14.

Perez J, et al. (2000). Altered cAMP-dependent protein kinase A in platelets of patients with obsessive–compulsive disorder. Am J Psychiatry. **157**: 284–6.

Phillips KA, et al. (2010). Should an obsessive–compulsive spectrum grouping of disorders be included in DSM-V? Depress Anxiety. **27**: 528–55.

Purcell R, et al. (1998a). Cognitive deficits in obsessive–compulsive disorder on tests of frontal-striatal function. Biol Psychiatry. **43**: 348–57.

Purcell R, et al. (1998b). Neuropsychological deficits in obsessive–compulsive disorder: a comparison with unipolar depression, panic disorder, and normal controls. Arch Gen Psychiatry. **55**: 415–23.

Rapoport JL, et al. (1992). Drug treatment of canine acral lick. Arch Gen Psychiatry. **48**: 517–21.

Rauch SL and Baxter LRJ (1998). Neuroimaging in obsessive–compulsive disorder and related disorders. In: Jenicke MA, Baer L, Minichiello WE, eds. Obsessive–Compulsive Disorders: Practical Management, 3rd edn. St Louis: Mosby.

Rauch SL, et al. (2000). Volume reduction in the caudate nucleus following stereotactic placement of lesions in the anterior cingulate cortex in humans: a morphometric magnetic resonance imaging study. J Neurosurg. **93**: 1019–25.

Rauch SL, et al. (2001). Probing striato-thalamic function in obsessive–compulsive disorder and Tourette syndrome using neuroimaging methods. Adv Neurol. **85**: 207–24.

Rauch SL, et al. (2004). What is the role of psychiatric neurosurgery in the 21st century? Revista Brasileira De Psiquiatria. **26**: 4–5.

Reimold M, et al. (2007). Reduced availability of serotonin transporters in obsessive–compulsive disorder correlates with symptom severity—a [11C]DASB PET study. J Neural Transm. **114**: 1603–9.

Ridley RM (1994). The psychology of perseverative and stereotyped behavior. Prog Neurobiol. **44**: 221–31.

Robbins TW (2007). Shifting and stopping: fronto-striatal substrates, neurochemical modulation and clinical implications. Philos Trans R Soc Lond B Biol Sci. **362**: 917–32.

Rosenberg DR and Keshavan MS (1998). Toward a neurodevelopmental model of obsessive–compulsive disorder. Biol Psychiatry. **43**: 623–40.

Rosenberg DR, et al. (2000). Decrease in caudate glutamate concentration in pediatric obsessive–compulsive disorder patients taking paroxetine. J Am Acad Child Adolesc Psychiatry. **39**: 1096–103.

Rosenberg DR, et al. (2001). Brain anatomy and chemistry may predict treatment response in paediatric obsessive–compulsive disorder. Int J Neuropsychopharmacol. **4**: 179–90.

Rosenberg DR, et al. (2004). Reduced anterior cingulate glutamatergic concentrations in childhood OCD and major depression versus healthy controls. J Am Acad Child Adolesc Psychiatry. **43**: 1146–53.

Saint-Cyr JA, et al. (1995). Behavior and the basal ganglia. In: Weiner WJ, Lang AE, eds. Behavioral Neurology of Movement Disorders. New York: Raven Press.

Sampaio AS, et al. (2013). Genetic association studies in obsessive–compulsive disorder. Rev Psiq Clin. **40**: 177–90.

Saxena S, et al. (2004). Cerebral glucose metabolism in obsessive–compulsive hoarding. Am J Psychiatry. **161**: 1038–48.

Shapira NA, *et al.* (2003). Brain activation by disgust-inducing pictures in obsessive–compulsive disorder. *Biol Psychiatry.* **54**: 751–6.

Shugart YY, *et al.* (2006). Genomewide linkage scan for obsessive–compulsive disorder: evidence for suscep-tibility loci on chromosomes 3q, 7p, 1q, 15q, and 6q. *Mol Psychiatry.* **11**: 763–70.

Simpson HB, *et al.* (2003). Serotonin transporters in obsessive–compulsive disorder: a positron emission tomography study with [(11) C] McN 5652. *Biol Psychiatry.* **54**: 1414–21.

Singer HS, *et al.* (2012). Moving from PANDAS to CANS. *J Pediatr.* **160**: 725–31.

Snider LA, *et al.* (2005). Antibiotic prophylaxis with azithromycin or penicillin for childhood-onset neuropsy-chiatric disorders. *Biol Psychiat.* **57**: 788–92.

Stein DJ (1999). Single photon emission computed tomography of the brain with tc-99m HMPAO during sumatriptan challenge in obsessive–compulsive disorder: investigating the functional role of the serotonin auto-receptor. *Prog Neuropsychopharmacol Biol Psychiat.* **23**: 1079–99.

Stein DJ (2002). Seminar on obsessive–compulsive disorder. *Lancet.* **360**: 397–405.

Stein DJ, *et al.* (1994). Neuropsychiatry of obsessive–compulsive disorder. In: Hollander E, Zohar J, Marazziti D, Olivier B, eds. *Current Insights in Obsessive–Compulsive Disorder.* Chichester: Wiley.

Stein DJ, *et al.* (2000). The cognitive-affective neuroscience of obsessive–compulsive disorder. *Curr Psychiat Rep.* **2**: 341–6.

Stein DJ, *et al.* (2001). The psychobiology of obsessive–compulsive disorder: how important is the role of disgust? *Curr Psychiat Rep.* **3**: 281–7.

Stern L, *et al.* (1998). Treatment of severe, drug resistant obsessive compulsive disorder with the 5HT1D agonist sumatriptan. *Eur Neuropsychopharmacol.* **8**: 325–8.

Stewart SE, *et al.* (2013). Genome-wide association study of obsessive–compulsive disorder. *Mol Psychiatry.* **18**: 788–98.

Swedo SE and Grant PJ (2005). Annotation: PANDAS: a model for human autoimmune disease. *J Child Psychol Psychiat Allied Discipl.* **46**: 227–34.

Swedo SE, *et al.* (1989). High prevalence of obsessive–compulsive symptoms in patients with Sydenham's chorea. *Am J Psychiatry.* **146**: 246–9.

Swedo SE, *et al.* (1998). Pediatric autoimmune neuropsychiatric disorders associated with streptococcal infections: clinical description of the first 50 cases. *Am J Psychiatry.* **155**: 264–71.

Swedo SE, Leckman JF, and Rose NR. (2012). From Research Subgroup to Clinical Syndrome: Modifying the PANDAS Criteria to Describe PANS (Pediatric Acute-onset Neuropsychiatric Syndrome). *Pediatr Therapeut.* **2**: 113.

Szeszko PR, *et al.* (1999). Orbital frontal and amygdala volume reductions in obsessive–compulsive disorder. *Arch Gen Psychiatry.* **56**: 913–19.

Talbot PS (2004). The molecular neuroimaging of anxiety disorders. *Curr Psychiat Rep.* **6**: 274–9.

Taylor S (2013). Molecular genetics of obsessive–compulsive disorder: a comprehensive meta-analysis of genetic association studies. *Mol Psychiatry.* **18**: 799–805.

Thoren P, *et al.* (1980). Clomipramine treatment of obsessive–compulsive disorder. II. Biochemical aspects. *Arch Gen Psychiatry.* **37**: 1289–94.

Urraca N, *et al.* (2004). Mu opioid receptor gene as a candidate for the study of obsessive–compulsive disorder with and without tics. *Am J Med Genet.* **B127**: 94–6.

van der Wee NJ, *et al.* (2004). Enhanced dopamine transporter density in psychotropic-naive patients with obsessive–compulsive disorder shown by [123I] beta -CIT SPECT. *Am J Psychiatry.* **161**: 2201 6.

van Grootheest DS, *et al.* (2005). Twin studies on obsessive–compulsive disorder: a review. *Twin Res Hum Genet.* **8**: 450–8.

Walitza S, *et al.* (2010). Genetics of early-onset obsessive–compulsive disorder. *Eur Child Adolesc Psychiatry.* **19**: 227–35.

Whiteside SP, *et al.* (2004). A meta-analysis of functional neuroimaging in obsessive–compulsive disorder. *Psychiat Res.* **132**: 69–79.

Whiteside SP, *et al.* (2006). A magnetic resonance spectroscopy investigation of obsessive–compulsive dis-order and anxiety. *Psychiatry Res.* **146**: 137–47.

Williams KE and Koran LM (1997). Obsessive–compulsive disorder in pregnancy, the puerperium, and the premenstruum. *J Clin Psychiatry.* **58**: 330–4.

Zai G, et al. (2004). Myelin oligodendrocyte glycoprotein (MOG) gene is associated with obsessive–compulsive disorder. *Am J Med Genet.* **B129**: 64–8.

Zai G, et al. (2005). Evidence for the gamma-amino-butyric acid type B receptor 1 (GABBR1) gene as a susceptibility factor in obsessive–compulsive disorder. *Am J Med Genet.* **134**: 25–9.

Zald DH and Kim SW (1996). Anatomy and function of the orbital frontal cortex, I: anatomy, neurocircuitry, and obsessive–compulsive disorder. *J Neuropsychiat Clin Neurosci.* **8**: 125–38.

Zohar J and Insel TR (1987). Drug treatment of obsessive–compulsive disorder. *J Affect Disord* **13**: 193–202.

Zohar J, et al. (1988). Serotonergic responsivity in obsessive–compulsive disorder: effects of chronic clomi-pramine treatment. *Arch Gen Psychiatry.* **45**: 167–72.

Zuchner S, et al. (2006). SLITRK1 mutations in trichotillomania. *Mol Psychiatry.* **11**: 888–9.

Zungu-Dirwayi N, et al. (1999). Are musical obsessions a temporal lobe phenomenon? *J Neuropsychiat Clin Neurosci.* **11**: 398–400.

# Further reading

Figee M, de Koning P, and Klaassen S (2014). Deep brain stimulation induces striatal dopamine release in obsessive–compulsive disorder. *Biol Psychiatry.* **75**: 647–52.

Burguiere E, Monteiro P, Mallet L, Feng G and Graybiel AM (2015). Striatal circuits, habits, and implications for obsessive–compulsive disorder. Current Opinion in Neurobiology, **30**:59–65

Chamberlain SR, et al. (2008). Orbitofrontal dysfunction in patients with obsessive–compulsive disorder and their unaffected relatives. *Science.* **18**; 321: 421–2.

Pauls DL (2012) The Genetics of obsessive–compulsive disorder: current status. In: Zohar J, ed. *Obsessive–Compulsive Disorder—Current Science and Clinical Practice.* World Psychiatric Association, Wiley-Blackwell. pp. 277–99.

Pooley EC, Fineberg N, and Harrison PJ (2007). The met[158] allele of catechol-O-methyltransferase (COMT) is associated with obsessive–compulsive disorder in men: case-control study and meta-analysis. *Mol Psychiatry.* **12**, 556–61.

# Chapter 4

# Pharmacotherapy and somatic treatments

## Key points

- First-line treatment for OCD should be with SSRIs for most cases.
- The treatment effect in OCD may emerge slowly and gradually over weeks and months.
- Long-term treatment in OCD protects against relapse.
- Pharmacotherapy strategies for SRI-resistant OCD are under investigation; data mostly suggest a role for low-dose D2 blockers as augmentation treatment.
- First-line pharmacotherapy for some obsessive-compulsive and related disorders, such as BDD, is similar to that for OCD.
- First-line pharmacotherapy for some obsessive-compulsive and related disorders, such as trichotillomania, differs from that for OCD.

## 4.1 The pharmacological specificity of obsessive-compulsive disorder

The weight of evidence shows that OCD responds preferentially to drugs which powerfully inhibit the synaptic reuptake of serotonin (SRIs). These are the:

- Tricyclic antidepressant clomipramine;
- More highly selective serotonin reuptake inhibitors (SSRIs).

RCTs have shown that these drugs are clinically efficacious treatments for OCD, both in the presence and absence of comorbid depression (reviewed in Fineberg et al. 2012; Fineberg and Gale 2005). In contrast, despite occasional positive trials, other classes of medication (monoamine oxidase inhibitors, benzodiazepines, dopamine blockers) have not consistently been found efficacious (Table 4.1). This selective pharmacological response has generated hypotheses about the role of serotonin in the aetiology of OCD, but, so far, no unifying theory has been proved (see Chapter 3), and the mechanisms by which SSRIs exert anti-obsessional benefits remain only partially understood (Fineberg et al. 1997; Fineberg et al. 2012).

## 4.2 Clomipramine

Building on several small positive trials (reviewed in Fineberg and Gale 2005), two seminal multicentre studies of clomipramine for non-depressed adult patients with OCD (Clomipramine Collaborative Study Group 1991; de Veaugh-Geiss et al. 1989) and one for childhood OCD (De Veaugh-Geiss et al. 1992) were performed early on. Significant differences between drug and placebo emerged in favour of clomipramine as early as the first week of treatment. However, the benefits of clomipramine, given in flexible doses, continued to increase slowly and gradually over several weeks.

| Table 4.1 The pharmacological specificity of OCD | |
|---|---|
| Effective | Ineffective |
| • Potent SRIs, e.g.:<br>  • clomipramine<br>  • fluvoxamine<br>  • fluoxetine<br>  • sertraline<br>  • paroxetine<br>  • citalopram<br>  • escitalopram | • Tricyclics (apart from clomipramine)<br>• Monoamine oxidase inhibitors<br>• Lithium<br>• Benzodiazepines<br>• Buspirone<br>• Electroconvulsive therapy |

Potentially effective in combination with SRIs:
• First-generation antipsychotics, e.g. haloperidol
• Second-generation antipsychotics, e.g. olanzapine, quetiapine, risperidone, aripiprazole.

(Reproduced from *Aust NZ J Psychiatry*, **47**(2), Fineberg NA et al., Pharmacotherapy of obsessive-compulsive disorder: evidence base and beyond, p. 121–41, Copyright (2013), with permission from Sage Publications.)

# 4.3 **Selective serotonin reuptake inhibitors**

The introduction of SSRIs provided the potential for agents that were not only efficacious for OCD, but that also had a superior safety and tolerability profile to clomipramine. The efficacy of fluvoxamine, sertraline, fluoxetine, paroxetine, citalopram, and escitalopram in the treatment of OCD has been demonstrated unequivocally in large-scale acute-phase studies (described in detail in the following sections). Several SSRIs have also been shown effective in paediatric OCD, some from the age of 7 years onwards. Like clomipramine, the treatment effect increases gradually over many weeks. Although clomipramine is a powerful SRI, it has an active metabolite with strong noradrenergic properties. That the more highly selective SSRIs are also beneficial, showing a similar incremental effect, suggests that their anti-obsessional actions are related to their SRI properties.

## 4.3.1 **Placebo-controlled trials of fluvoxamine**

### 4.3.1.1 *Adults*

Small double-blind studies, some employing a crossover design (Perse et al. 1987), demonstrated similar efficacy in depressed and non-depressed OCD patients (Goodman et al. 1989; Jenike et al. 1990a). In the study by Cottraux et al. (1990), fluvoxamine also showed superiority over placebo, in spite of concurrent exposure therapy in the placebo group. The multicentre placebo-controlled study by Goodman et al. (1996) confirmed superiority for fluvoxamine (100–300 mg). Obsessions and compulsions both improved, with a possible earlier benefit for obsessions. Another multicentre study demonstrated efficacy for controlled-release (CR) fluvoxamine (100–300 mg) (Hollander et al. 2003a).

### 4.3.1.2 *Children*

Riddle et al. (2001) demonstrated efficacy for fluvoxamine (50–200 mg) in 120 children aged 8–17 years. Only three patients on fluvoxamine and one on placebo withdrew through adverse effects. This finding suggests efficacy and tolerability for fluvoxamine in childhood OCD. Anecdotal data indicate, however, that some paediatric patients, perhaps particularly those with impulsive or tic disorders, may develop behavioural disinhibition after fluvoxamine (Harris et al. 2010).

### 4.3.2 **Placebo-controlled trials of sertraline**

4.3.2.1 *Adults*

Placebo-controlled studies by Chouinard *et al.* (1990) and Kronig *et al.* (1999), and a multicentre trial by Greist *et al.* (1995a) demonstrated efficacy for sertraline in daily doses ranging from 50 to 200 mg. Jenike *et al.* (1990b) found no group differences in a study that was arguably underpowered.

4.3.2.2 *Children*

March *et al.* (1998) found a significant advantage over placebo for sertraline, titrated up to 200 mg, in a cohort of children and adolescents. Cardiovascular parameters showed no clinically meaningful abnormalities. Although insomnia, nausea, agitation, and tremor occurred more often in the drug-treated group, only 13% of sertraline patients discontinued early because of adverse effects (compared with 3% placebo), suggesting that sertraline is safe up to doses of 200 mg in children (Wilens *et al.* 1999). In the Pediatric OCD Treatment Study (POTS 2004), 112 children and adolescents received CBT alone, sertraline alone, combined CBT and sertraline, or pill placebo. All three active treatments appeared acceptable and well tolerated, with no evidence of treatment-emergent harm to self or to others. The lack of a matched control treatment for CBT limited conclusions about relative efficacy; sertraline alone, and in combination with CBT, was efficacious, compared with pill placebo.

A pooled analysis of the childhood OCD studies, comparing 'numbers needed to treat' with those 'needed to harm', revealed no suicidal actions and a positive risk ratio for the use of sertraline in children and adolescents with OCD (March *et al.* 2006).

### 4.3.3 **Placebo-controlled trials of fluoxetine**

4.3.3.1 *Adults*

Two multicentre studies benefited from a design that allowed comparison of different fixed doses. In the study by Montgomery *et al.* (1993), the 20 mg dose fared no better than placebo, while the 40 mg dose and the 60 mg dose were superior. In the larger, longer study by Tollefson *et al.* (1994), all fixed doses of fluoxetine emerged as superior to placebo, but there was a trend toward superiority for the 60 mg dose. In a placebo-controlled active comparator study (Jenike *et al.* 1997), fluoxetine was superior to placebo and also to the monoamine oxidase inhibitor phenelzine, which did not differentiate from placebo.

4.3.3.2 *Children*

Three studies have looked at fluoxetine in childhood OCD, all showing superiority over placebo. Riddle *et al.*'s crossover study (1992) used fixed doses of 20 mg. Behavioural activation occurred as an adverse effect in a few children, and one left the study early because of suicidal ideation. The authors considered these side effects to be dose-related and advocated initiating treatment at doses lower than 20 mg/day. Geller *et al.* (2001) took a larger cohort, titrating doses upwards from 10 mg to 60 mg over 13 weeks. Fluoxetine was superior to placebo and well tolerated, with similar dropout rates from adverse events on drug and placebo. In the trial by Leibowitz *et al.* (2002), the dose range was extended to 80 mg after the first 6 weeks. After 8 weeks, responders could continue double-blind treatment for a further 8 weeks. No patient withdrew from adverse effects. These results suggest fluoxetine is a generally safe and effective treatment for children and adolescents with OCD. However, its full effect may take more than 8 weeks to develop.

### 4.3.4 **Placebo-controlled trials of paroxetine**

4.3.4.1 *Adults*

The multicentre study by Zohar and Judge (1996) included clomipramine as a comparator agent. Paroxetine, given in doses up to 60 mg, was significantly more effective than placebo and of comparable efficacy to clomipramine (50–250 mg). In another large trial, Hollander et al. (2003b) tested paroxetine in fixed doses (20 mg, 40 mg, and 60 mg) against placebo. Both higher doses significantly outperformed both placebo and the 20 mg dose which did not separate from placebo. The comparator study by Stein et al. (2007), which was extended up to 24 weeks, included a 40 mg fixed-dose arm which showed efficacy against placebo at the 12- and 24-week rating points.

### 4.3.4.2 *Children*

Geller et al. (2004) reported efficacy for paroxetine (10–50 mg) in a study of 204 children and adolescents from as young as 7 years. Paroxetine was generally well tolerated; 10.2% of patients in the paroxetine group and 2.9% in the placebo group discontinued treatment because of adverse events.

## 4.3.5 **Placebo-controlled trials of citalopram**

### 4.3.5.1 *Adults*

The multinational placebo-controlled study by Montgomery et al. (2001) showed efficacy for fixed doses of 20 mg, 40 mg, and 60 mg of citalopram, compared with placebo. Citalopram was well tolerated and improved psychosocial disability on the Sheehan Disability Scale (Sheehan et al. 1996).

## 4.3.6 **Placebo-controlled studies of escitalopram**

### 4.3.6.1 *Adults*

Escitalopram, an SSRI with dual actions on the SERT (Sanchez et al. 2004), was investigated in a multicentre, active-referenced study which extended for as long as 24 weeks (Stein et al. 2007). Patients were randomized to escitalopram 10 mg/day, escitalopram 20 mg/day, paroxetine 40 mg/day, or placebo. After 12 weeks, both 20 mg escitalopram and paroxetine were superior to placebo, and, by week 24, all three active treatments were superior. These results highlight the importance of continuing treatment beyond the acute phase. They suggest escitalopram (10–20 mg) is efficacious, with a faster onset of action for the 20 mg dose.

## 4.3.7 **Which serotonin reuptake inhibitor is most clinically effective?**

Clinical effectiveness usually depends upon a balance between efficacy, safety, and tolerability.

| Practice point: when deciding upon a drug treatment … |
|---|
| Consider efficacy, safety, and tolerability. |

So far, only three controlled studies have compared the clinical effectiveness of different SSRIs, and the results were not strong enough to support the superior efficacy of any one compound (Bergeron et al. 2001; Mundo et al. 1997; Stein et al. 2007).

SSRIs are generally safe and well tolerated, according to the placebo-referenced treatment trials which reported adverse event-related withdrawal rates of around 5–15%. As a group, SSRIs cause unwanted nausea, insomnia, somnolence, dizziness, and diarrhoea. Sexual side effects include reduced libido and delayed orgasm, and they can also affect up to 30% of individuals (Monteiro et al. 1987).

When choosing a particular SSRI, the clinician should take account of pharmacokinetic variation which may result in unwanted interactions with other drugs being prescribed. In this respect, fluoxetine, paroxetine, and, to a much lesser extent, sertraline inhibit the P450 isoenzyme CYP 2D6 which metabolizes tricyclic antidepressants, antipsychotics, anti-arrhythmics, and beta-blockers, whereas fluvoxamine inhibits both CYP 1A2 and CYP 3A4, which eliminate warfarin, tricyclics, benzodiazepines, and some anti-arrhythmics. Citalopram and escitalopram are relatively free from hepatic interactions. Fluoxetine has a long half-life and fewer

**Table 4.2** Controlled studies comparing SSRIs with clomipramine (CMI)

| Drug and study | n | Design | Outcome | |
|---|---|---|---|---|
| | | | Efficacy | Tolerability |
| *Fluoxetine (FLX)* | | | | |
| Pigott et al. (1990) | 11 | CMI (50–250 mg) vs FLX (20–80 mg) | CMI = FLX | FLX > CMI |
| Lopez-Ibor et al. (1996) | 30 vs 24 | CMI 150 mg vs FLX 40 mg | CMI = FLX on primary criterion | FLX = CMI |
| | | | CMI > FLX on other criteria | |
| *Fluvoxamine (FLV)* | | | | |
| Smeraldi et al. (1992) | 10 | CMI 200 mg vs FLV 200 mg | CMI = FLV | FLV = CMI |
| Freeman et al. (1994) | 30 vs 34 | CMI (150–250 mg) vs FLV (150–250 mg) | CMI = FLV | FLV > CMI (on severe effects) |
| Koran et al. (1996) | 42 vs 37 | CMI (100–250 mg) vs FLV (100–250 mg) | CMI = FLV | FLV = CMI |
| Milanfranchi et al. (1997) | 13 vs 13 | CMI (50–300 mg) vs FLV (50–300 mg) | CMI = FLV | FLV = CMI |
| Rouillon (1998) | 105 vs 112 | CMI (150–300 mg) vs FLV (150–300 mg) | CMI = FLV | FLV > CMI |
| *Paroxetine (PAR)* | | | | |
| Zohar and Judge (1996) | 99 vs 201 vs 99 | CMI (50–250 mg) vs PAR (20–60 mg) vs placebo | CMI > placebo | PAR > CMI |
| | | | PAR > placebo | |
| *Sertraline (SER)* | | | | |
| Bisserbe et al. (1997) | 82 vs 86 | CMI (50–200 mg) vs SER (50–200 mg) | SER = CMI | SER > CMI |

discontinuation effects, which can be advantageous for patients who forget to take their tablets. It has also been extensively used in pregnancy and generally shown to be safe (Bairy et al. 2007).

Head-to-head studies have demonstrated that, whereas the SRIs appear equally efficacious in treating OCD, SSRIs are tolerated better than clomipramine (Table 4.2). For example, in the study of Zohar and Judge (1996), the dropout rate from adverse effects on clomipramine (17%) was higher than for paroxetine (9%). Rouillon (1998) also reported that clomipramine was associated with significantly more withdrawals associated with side effects than fluvoxamine, and, in the analysis by Bisserbe et al. (1997), superior tolerability of sertraline over clomipramine produced a greater overall benefit.

Clomipramine can also be associated with potentially dangerous side effects. Cardiotoxicity and cognitive impairment occur substantially more with clomipramine than with SSRIs. In addition there is an increased risk of convulsions in patients taking clomipramine (up to 2%). Overdose on clomipramine can prove fatal, and this needs to be borne in mind when prescribing for OCD, in view of the elevated suicide risk associated with the illness. Clomipramine is also associated with greater impairment of sexual performance (up to 80% of patients), compared with SSRIs (up to 30% of patients) (Monteiro et al. 1987), weight gain (Maina et al. 2003a), and troublesome anticholinergic effects. On the other hand, SSRIs are associated with initially increased nausea, agitation, and insomnia. The recent demonstration of prolongation of the electrocardiographic (ECG) QT interval associated with higher dose levels of citalopram (and, to a lesser extent, escitalopram) (US Food and Drug Administration 2012) argues for a degree of caution in using higher doses of these compounds in OCD, especially if individuals are taking other medications that increase the QT interval. However, a recent large study found no elevated risks of ventricular arrhythmia or all-cause, cardiac, or non-cardiac mortality associated with citalopram doses exceeding 40 mg/day (Zivin et al. 2013).

### 4.3.8 Suicide in children with obsessive-compulsive disorder receiving selective serotonin reuptake inhibitors

Meta-analyses (for a definition, see Section 4.3.9) examining the effects of SSRIs in children aged 6–18 years have been performed, following warnings from the American Food and Drug Administration that SSRIs in the young may increase the risk of suicidal thoughts and behaviours. In the study by Bridge et al. (2007), 27 RCTs of SSRIs, of which six were in OCD, were identified. There were no completed suicides. The pooled absolute rates of either suicidal ideation/suicide attempt (treatment vs placebo) in OCD (1% vs 0.3%) compared favourably with the pooled absolute clinical response rates (treatment vs placebo, 52% vs 32%). The authors concluded that the benefits of SSRIs probably outweigh the risks in the OCD paediatric population. March et al. (2006) calculated the number needed to treat (NNT) and number needed to harm (NNH) for multicentre trials of sertraline in children and adolescents with major depressive disorder and OCD. The NNT ranged from 2 to 10, with no apparent age effect in OCD. No patients reported suicidality in the two OCD trials, giving a NNH approaching infinity. The authors concluded a positive benefit-to-risk ratio for sertraline in paediatric OCD.

---

Practice points: when choosing an SRI for OCD...

- Use an SSRI as first line for most cases.
- Check for potential drug interactions, and select SSRI accordingly.
- Check for potential suicidal behaviour.
- Choose clomipramine for those who fail treatment with SSRIs or who cannot tolerate them.

### 4.3.9 **Meta-analyses of serotonin reuptake inhibitors**

Meta-analyses combine data from separate studies, using specific statistical techniques. They can provide a more objective and quantifiable measure of treatment effect size than narrative reviews. However, they are subject to the confounding effects of imbalances in populations studied, differing severities, and differing methodology for each study, so results for analyses on the OCD trials, which spanned several decades, must be viewed with a great deal of caution (Watson and Rees 2008). There is also the risk that a significant difference reported in a large meta-analysis may reflect only a small difference between the treatments, which may not be clinically relevant. For these reasons, the evidence from meta-analyses is considered weaker than evidence from individual controlled studies. In short, meta-analyses cannot substitute for high-quality head-to-head comparator trials.

Meta-analysis of OCD trials introduced the idea that less 'serotonin-selective' agents, such as clomipramine, might have a greater effect size than SSRIs; whereas most meta-analyses demonstrated significant advantages for all SRIs over placebo, some showed superiority for clomipramine over SSRIs which were more or less comparable (Abramowitz 1997; Ackerman and Greenland 2002; Greist et al. 1995b; Jenike et al. 1990a; Kobak et al. 1998; Piccinelli et al. 1995; Stein et al. 1995). Variation between individual studies in factors, such as year of publication, length of single-blind pre-randomization period, length of trial, severity of OCD, and the recent rise in placebo response rates, were acknowledged to have potentially biased the results in favour of clomipramine.

The UK National Collaborating Centre for Mental Health systematically accessed unpublished, as well as published, randomized studies, which were included in their meta-analysis only if they met stringent methodological criteria, as part of the UK National Institute for Health and Care Excellence (NICE) comprehensive treatment guideline (NICE 2006). Clomipramine and SSRIs could not be distinguished, in terms of efficacy, whereas there was some limited evidence suggesting that clomipramine was associated with a higher rate of adverse event-related premature trial discontinuations than SSRIs (<https://www.nice.org.uk>).

Geller et al. (2003a) performed a meta-analysis on pharmacotherapy for childhood OCD. The results were consistent with the adult literature. In the absence of head-to–head studies, the authors recommended that clomipramine should not generally be used first-line in children because of its more problematic side effect profile. Fineberg et al. (2004) directly compared SRI treatment trials in childhood OCD with those in adult OCD in a meta-analysis. Effect sizes overlapped for children and adults, to the extent that it was not possible to discriminate between the efficacy and tolerability of SRIs in children and adults with OCD. These results imply a similar treatment response for childhood and adulthood OCD.

### 4.3.10 **Which dose?**

Dose finding studies have suggested that higher doses (20 mg escitalopram; 60 mg citalopram, fluoxetine, paroxetine; 200 mg sertraline) are more effective, although the evidence for higher doses of sertraline and citalopram was less clear-cut (reviewed in Fineberg et al. 2012). Clomipramine and fluvoxamine have not been investigated using fixed-dose comparator groups. The study by Montgomery (1980) did show efficacy for a relatively low fixed dose of 75 mg clomipramine. A meta-analysis that used weighted mean difference to examine the mean change in Y-BOCS score and pooled absolute risk difference to examine dichotomous outcomes found that, compared with either low or medium doses, higher doses of SSRIs were associated with improved treatment efficacy, using either the Y-BOCS score or the proportion of treatment responders as an outcome (Bloch et al. 2010). The dose of an SSRI was not associated with the number of all-cause dropouts. However, a higher dose of an SSRI was associated with a significantly higher proportion of dropouts due to side effects. These results suggest that higher doses of SSRIs are associated with greater efficacy in the treatment of OCD that is somewhat counterbalanced by the greater side effect burden. This SSRI efficacy

| Table 4.3 Recommended dose ranges of SSRIs for adult OCD* | |
|---|---|
| Medication | Dose range |
| ªCitalopram | 20–60 mg/day |
| ªEscitalopram | 10–20 mg/day |
| Fluoxetine | 20–80 mg/day |
| Fluvoxamine | 50–300 mg/day |
| Paroxetine | 20–60 mg/day |
| Sertraline | 50–200 mg/day |

* For children and adolescents (aged 8–16 years), starting at half the lowest listed dose is advisable. Lower doses than those listed are usually recommended in the elderly.

ª Doses above 40 mg citalopram and 20 mg escitalopram in adults exceed the licensed limit in some countries and may be associated with ECG changes.

pattern stands in contrast to other psychiatric disorders like major depressive disorder (Bloch *et al.* 2010). Table 4.3 shows recommended dose ranges for SSRIs in OCD.

### 4.3.11 **Dose titration**

Fast upwards titration may produce earlier responses, but the long-term benefits of this approach are unclear. A single-blind study compared rapid dose escalation with sertraline to 150 mg over 5 days with slower dose escalation over 15 days, and found an early advantage for the rapid titration group which disappeared after week 6 (Bogetto *et al.* 2002). In another study, pulse loading with intravenous clomipramine produced a large and rapid decrease in obsessive symptoms, but oral pulse loading did not, and the early advantages were not sustained over treatment (Koran *et al.* 1997). In contrast, the escitalopram dose finding study (Stein *et al.* 2007) showed that, although slower than the 20 mg dose, the 10 mg dose eventually did reach efficacy after 24 weeks.

The arguments for slower dose increases are persuasive, particularly in children and the elderly. Early SSRI-related adverse effects, such as nausea and agitation, can be ameliorated by slowly titrating upwards over weeks and months. Particular care with higher doses is required for cases with comorbidity. For example, patients with comorbid panic disorder may be particularly sensitive to early anxiogenic effects of SSRIs, and lower-than-average doses may be required for the first week or two. Those with bipolar disorder are susceptible to switching into mania and may require additional mood stabilizers. Longer-term side effects, such as sleep disturbance and headache, are also dose-related and need to be monitored. Sexual dysfunction is a common cause of drug discontinuation, and, if necessary, strategies, such as dose reduction, switch to another SSRI, switch to a non-SSRI, short drug holidays, or use of drugs with restorative potency (e.g. sildenafil, mianserin, buspirone (Aizenberg *et al.* 1999) (Hirsch and Birnbaum 2013), can be considered in stable cases.

### 4.3.12 **The response to serotonin reuptake inhibitors is slow and gradual**

Patients should be warned, at the outset of treatment with clomipramine or an SSRI, that the anti-obsessional effect takes several weeks to develop fully. Sometimes, progress seems remarkably slow, and patients may find it difficult to acknowledge changes are occurring. It may be helpful to recruit family or friends to substantiate these improvements.

Side effects, such as nausea and agitation, tend to emerge early, before signs of improvement are consolidated, but usually abate over time. However, placebo-referenced gains accrue for at least 6 months (Stein et al. 2007) and, according to open-label follow-up data, for at least 2 years (Rasmussen et al. 1997). It is important therefore to allow time for the treatment effect to develop and not to discontinue or change the drug prematurely. In the absence of reliable early predictors of response, a trial of at least 12 weeks at the maximum tolerated dose and careful assessment is advisable before judging its efficacy. Although response to medication does not necessarily imply symptom remission, it is usually associated with significant improvement in the quality of life (Hollander et al. 2010; Stein et al. 2007; Tenney et al. 2003).

### 4.3.13 Response and remission on serotonin reuptake inhibitor treatment

The response to treatment with an SRI is characteristically partial, at least in the early stages. Early work suggested that reduction in Y-BOCS scores of around 25% from baseline represents a clinically relevant improvement, although more recent work indicates that this is a fairly conservative target. In placebo-controlled trials, between 30% and 60% of cases reached this level of clinical response within the acute treatment phase (Fineberg and Gale 2005). However, it is important to recognize that the patients studied in RCTs are often drawn from centres specializing in OCD, which results in lower response rates because more treatment-resistant patients are seen at such sites. Open-label studies are usually associated with higher rates of SRI response than placebo trials, because all patients know they are receiving active treatment.

---

**Practice points: when starting treatment with an SRI...**

- Check for comorbidity that might impact on the initial dose.
- For most adult patients, start treatment with average doses (children and adolescents start with lower doses).
- Advise the patient that the treatment effect comes on slowly and that many side effects will abate with time.
- Recruit family member or friend to help assess treatment response.
- Increase dose gradually, at intervals of several weeks, titrating upwards against clinical response, to maximal doses.
- Continue for at least 12 weeks before judging efficacy.
- Remission and recovery are potentially achievable goals.

---

The concept of remission for OCD is more debatable, and there is no universally accepted definition. It has been described as a brief period, during which sufficient improvement has occurred that the individual no longer suffers with OCD, while recovery represents a long-lasting remission (Simpson et al. 2006). Studies have chosen remission criteria, ranging from Y-BOCS ≤16 to Y-BOCS ≤7, and have demonstrated that remission can be achieved on SSRI in up to 50% of cases (Simpson et al. 2006; Stein et al. 2007).

### 4.3.14 What if patients do not respond on serotonin reuptake inhibitors?

#### 4.3.14.1 *Review diagnosis and compliance*

Failure to respond should alert the clinician to the possibility of misdiagnosis. Tourette's syndrome and Asperger's syndrome are just two OCD spectrum disorders that can easily be mistaken for OCD, while alcohol abuse may be hidden. Adherence to the drug regimen should also be confirmed. It can be helpful to measure drug plasma levels. For example, rapid metabolizers of SRIs might respond less well. It is not clear how common a problem this

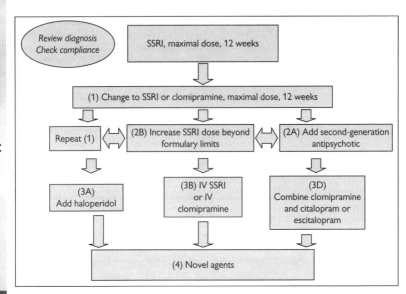

Figure 4.1 SRI-resistant OCD: a treatment algorithm.

might be in the OCD population. For patients with OCD, various negative clinical predictors have been described, including hoarding symptoms, comorbid tics, and schizotypal personality disorder—consistent with evidence that the dopamine system is important in their mediation.

Following poor response to an adequate trial of an SRI, the clinician has a variety of options (Figure 4.1). The evidence supporting these approaches is not as strong as for first-line treatments and relies on small-scale trials. Switching to a different SSRI or clomipramine is the usual first step. Subsequently, one may consider adding an antipsychotic agent or elevating the dose of an SRI beyond formulary dose limits (perhaps particularly relevant when there has been a partial response). Alternative options include changing the mode of delivery or introducing novel agents. The clinician should weigh up the relative advantages and disadvantages of these approaches and discuss them with the patient before proceeding.

### 4.3.14.2 *Adding an antipsychotic*

For truly SRI-resistant cases, the strongest evidence supports adding low doses of dopamine blockers to existing SRI therapy; earlier placebo-controlled randomized trials were undertaken with first-generation antipsychotics, and more recent studies (reviewed in Fineberg et al. 2006b; Komossa et al. 2010), including meta-analyses (Dold et al. 2013; Fineberg et al. 2006a; Ipser et al. 2006), have confirmed the effectiveness of the better tolerated new-generation antipsychotic agents, such as olanzapine (5–10 mg/day), quetiapine (200–300 mg/day), risperidone (1–2mg/day), and aripiprazole (10–15 mg/day), in adults. In the meta-analysis by Dold et al. (2013), superior efficacy was observed for risperidone, compared with other second-generation antipsychotics. Another meta-regression analysis suggested that $D_2$ and $D_3$ dopamine receptor affinity predicts efficacy of antipsychotic drugs in OCD, with aripiprazole being a particularly good option (Ducasse et al. 2014). Another analysis (Bloch et al. 2006) concluded that SRI-refractory patients with comorbid tics responded particularly well to adding antipsychotics.

Head-to-head studies are ultimately needed to determine the relative efficacy of different antipsychotic agents and doses. We suggest starting with low doses (around 0.5 mg risperidone, 50 mg quetiapine) and titrating upwards gradually, monitoring for clinical response and side effects. We also need to establish reliable predictors of response to antipsychotic augmentation strategies. A history of fewer previously failed SRI trials and generally higher overall baseline scores for obsessions and compulsions, as well as counting/ordering and arranging compulsions, were found to predict response to adjunctive quetiapine (Carey et al. 2012). Other factors are, however, also likely to play an important role in predicting outcome.

Longer-term studies are also needed to clarify long-term efficacy and risks of metabolic side effects. Second-generation antipsychotics, such as risperidone and quetiapine, may currently be preferred as the first-line strategy, since they are generally well tolerated in the context of short-term efficacy trials. Weight gain and drowsiness have been reported in trials of olanzapine (Bystritsky et al. 2004) and quetiapine (Fineberg et al. 2005). It remains uncertain as to how long patients should remain on augmented treatment; a small retrospective study by Maina et al. (2003b) showed that the majority of patients who had responded to the addition of an antipsychotic to their SRI subsequently relapsed when the antipsychotic was withdrawn.

### 4.3.15 Increasing serotonin reuptake inhibitor dose above normal limits

#### 4.3.15.1 Selective serotonin reuptake inhibitor

Uncontrolled case reports suggest that individuals who have tolerated maximal doses of an SSRI without adverse reactions may benefit from further increasing SSRI doses above formulary limits without adverse effects developing, e.g. citalopram 160 mg/day (Bejerot and Bodlund 1998) and sertraline 400 mg/day (Byerly et al. 1996). The American Psychiatric Association guideline on treating OCD (Koran et al. 2007) provides a list of maximum doses that are occasionally prescribed. It is not yet possible to predict which individuals might respond best to this strategy. For 'fast metabolizers', or those who have failed to respond to conventional doses of an SSRI and are not experiencing adverse effects, the guideline (Koran and Simpson 2013; Koran et al. 2007) recommends 'occasionally prescribed' doses of up to 60 mg/day of escitalopram, 120 mg/day of fluoxetine, 450 mg/day of fluvoxamine, 100 mg/day of paroxetine, and 400 mg/day of sertraline. There would seem to be reasonable grounds for gradually and cautiously increasing daily doses of an SSRI if the patient is in good physical health, the SSRI is well tolerated, and plasma levels turn out to be low. Patients need to be advised that the proposed dose exceeds the usual recommended limits. It may be advisable to monitor cardiac conduction, e.g. by ECG monitoring, especially if prescribing high-dose citalopram or escitalopram. The elderly may also be susceptible to SSRI-induced electrolyte disturbances and bleeding tendencies, and, for those on anticoagulant therapy, especially if using high-dose fluoxetine, the international normalized ratio (INR) may require more stringent monitoring.

#### 4.3.15.2 Clomipramine

For clomipramine, doses up to 300 mg have been systematically investigated and found to be acceptable (De Veaugh-Geiss et al. 1989). However, given its propensity to produce anticholinergic side effects, a high risk of convulsions (up to 2%) and potentially dangerous cardiotoxicity, doses of clomipramine exceeding this level should usually be avoided, unless ECG and plasma level monitoring is available. Trough plasma levels of clomipramine combined with its metabolite desmethylclomipramine should usually be kept below 450 ng/mL to minimize toxicity (Szegedi et al. 1996).

#### 4.3.15.3 Intravenous clomipramine

Results from a controlled study support the use of intravenous clomipramine in adults resistant to oral treatment (Fallon et al. 1998), but this may not always be practical since on-hand resuscitation facilities are required. Intravenous infusions of citalopram, administered daily for 21 days, led to an early onset of response and was well tolerated and effective in an open trial in 39 outpatients who had failed two adequate trials of oral SRIs (Pallanti et al. 2002).

#### 4.3.15.4 *Serotonin reuptake inhibitor combinations*

Combinations of SRIs have been found useful in some studies (Diniz *et al.* 2011; Pallanti *et al.* 1999). However, caution is required if clomipramine is to be combined with SSRIs that potentially cross-react at the hepatic microsomes, and plasma level and ECG monitoring are usually recommended. Citalopram and escitalopram (and, to a lesser extent, sertraline) are less likely to interfere with the clearance of clomipramine and are therefore preferred for this approach.

#### 4.3.15.5 *Other compounds as monotherapy or augmentation agents*

A number of augmenting agents from various classes (e.g. lithium, buspirone, pindolol, inositol) have been studied in controlled trials in adulthood OCD, but, to date, findings have been negative or inconsistent.

Venlafaxine possesses significant SRI properties. In one study, venlafaxine was noted to be as effective as paroxetine (Denys *et al.* 2003), but, in other studies, it compared poorly with paroxetine (Denys *et al.* 2004) and clomipramine (Albert *et al.* 2002). Given the potential value of venlafaxine in treatment-resistant depression, there is an argument for a trial of this agent in patients with OCD and severe depression.

Mirtazapine as monotherapy has been reported to reduce the relapse rate in a placebo-controlled discontinuation study of OCD (Koran *et al.* 2005). Nevertheless, given the sparse data on mirtazapine, it is not considered as a first-line agent.

A randomized placebo-controlled trial of single-dose dexamfetamine produced short-lived benefits (Insel *et al.* 1983), while another RCT, comparing dexamfetamine and caffeine, noted that both compounds were associated with rapid improvement of obsessive-compulsive symptoms within a week (Koran *et al.* 2009), suggesting that stimulants, such as dexamfetamine, could play a role in treating OCD and may be considered in those with comorbid ADHD.

There is accruing evidence for the glutamatergic compounds ketamine (Bloch *et al.* 2012; Rodriguez *et al.* 2013), memantine, and riluzole in OCD. Memantine has been investigated as an adjunct to an SSRI in a few open-label trials and two small randomized placebo-controlled trials (Ghaleiha *et al.* 2013; Haghighi *et al.* 2013). Memantine has a relatively favourable profile in relation to tolerability and drug interaction. Preliminary results from open-label studies suggesting efficacy for riluzole (Coric *et al.* 2005), another glutamate-modulating agent, require substantiation in placebo-controlled trials.

Clonazepam may produce symptomatic benefit (Hewlett *et al.* 1992), possibly through improving associated anxiety. It may be less suitable in those with a previous history of benzodiazepine or other substance dependence. It has been suggested that antiepileptic mood stabilizers may, in combination with an SSRI, have a role in the treatment of OCD, but the supporting evidence at present is limited. Positive results were obtained in a small RCT of lamotrigine (a glutamate modulator) (Bruno *et al.* 2012) and another of topiramate (Berlin *et al.* 2010), in which the therapeutic effect was seen on reducing compulsions only. Adjunctive pregabalin has been investigated in an open-label case series only, with some signs of possible efficacy (Oulis *et al.* 2011), as has gabapentin (Corá-Locatelli *et al.* 1998).

## 4.4 Is long-term pharmacological treatment beneficial?

OCD is a chronic illness, and so treatment needs to keep the patient well over the longer term. A small number of double-blind studies, lasting up to 12 months, have shown that those who responded to acute treatment benefited from continuing with medication, with no evidence of tolerance developing. In the study by Tollefson *et al.* (1994), patients on all doses of fluoxetine (20, 40, and 60 mg) continued to improve, but additional significant improvements were evident for the 60 mg group only, suggesting added benefit for remaining at the higher dose level. In the larger extension study by Greist *et al.* (1995a), patients who had responded to 12 weeks' treatment with sertraline or placebo continued under double-blind conditions for 40 weeks. Improvements were sustained for those who remained on sertraline, and side effects improved over time. Fifty-nine completers were followed up for a further year on open-label sertraline and showed significant additional improvements in OCD symptoms over the course of the second year, with a reduced incidence of side effects, compared with the earlier study (Rasmussen *et al.* 1997).

### 4.4.1 How long should treatment continue?

One way of tackling this question is to explore whether continuation of treatment provides ongoing benefit and protects against relapse. Studies looking at the short-term effects of discontinuing clomipramine or SSRIs under double-blind, placebo-controlled conditions showed a rapid and incremental worsening of symptoms in people who switched to placebo (reviewed in Fineberg *et al.* 2012).

### 4.4.2 Relapse prevention trials

Relapse prevention studies are difficult to conduct, and the results of studies so far have been mixed, largely owing to methodological problems. The design involves selecting responders to an open-label drug and then randomizing them either to continuation or to placebo (Table 4.4). In the fluoxetine study by Romano *et al.* (2001), patients remaining on the highest dose (60 mg) showed significantly lower relapse rates (17.5%), implying an ongoing advantage for staying at the higher dose levels, but the study still did not discriminate between continuation of pooled fluoxetine and discontinuation. In spite of its larger size and longer duration, the study by Koran *et al.* (2002) was also unable to demonstrate a significant advantage for sertraline on the a priori criterion for preventing relapse—in this case, almost certainly because the criterion for relapse was too strictly defined. However, those remaining on sertraline showed significantly fewer 'dropouts due to relapse or insufficient clinical response' and 'acute exacerbation of symptoms', and ongoing sertraline was associated with continued improvement in Y-BOCS scores and quality of life measures. In a study of children and adolescents (Geller *et al.* 2003b), the overall relapse rate was not significantly higher in the placebo than paroxetine group (43.9% vs 34.7%), possibly because the duration of follow-up was too short. However, the large-scale study of paroxetine by Hollander *et al.* (2003b) clearly demonstrated a significantly better outcome for those remaining on the active drug over the 6-month double-blind discontinuation phase; 59% of patients randomized to placebo relapsed, compared with 38% remaining on paroxetine (20–60 mg), with paroxetine being well tolerated long-term. In another large relapse prevention study using escitalopram (10–20 mg), patients randomized to placebo relapsed significantly earlier. After 24 weeks, 52% of placebo cases had relapsed, compared with 24% on escitalopram, and the risk of relapsing on placebo was 2.7 times higher, compared with escitalopram (Fineberg *et al.* 2006c). Moreover, relapse per se, irrespective of treatment modality, was found to be associated with a significant loss of quality of life in multiple domains of psychosocial functioning, emphasizing the importance of remaining well (Hollander *et al.* 2010).

### 4.4.3 Relapse prevention as a treatment target

Taken together, these results suggest that relapse prevention is a desirable and realistic target for OCD treatment, and that continuation of SSRIs protects patients against relapse. This emphasizes the importance of maintaining treatment with medication at an effective dose level in the long term, i.e. for at least 12 months (NICE 2006), and argues against discontinuation of treatment, even after 1 year, if patients are doing well. The adage 'the dose that gets you well keeps you well' probably applies, and the possibility that some patients may retain response at

**Table 4.4** Double-blind studies of relapse prevention in OCD

| Study | Drug | Duration of prior drug treatment | n in discont. phase | Follow-up after discont. | Outcome |
|---|---|---|---|---|---|
| Bailer et al. (1995) | Paroxetine | 6 months | 44 | 24 weeks | Relapse rate on plac = parox Parox > plac on Y-BOCS |
| Romano et al. (1998) | Fluoxetine | 20 weeks | 71 | 52 weeks | Relapse rate on plac = pooled fluox Relapse rate on plac > fluox 60 mg |
| Koran et al. (2002) | Sertraline | 52 weeks | 223 | 28 weeks | Relapse rate on plac = sert Acute exacerb of OCD on plac > sert Dropout due to relapse on plac > sert |
| [a]Geller et al. (2003b) | Paroxetine | 16 weeks | 193 | 16 weeks | Relapse rate on plac = parox |
| Hollander et al. (2003b) | Paroxetine | 12 weeks | 105 | 36 weeks | Relapse rate on plac > parox |
| Fineberg et al. (2006c) | Escitalopram | 16 weeks | 322 | 24 weeks | Time to relapse on esc > plac Relapse rate on plac > esc |

[a] In children and adolescents.

a lower dose or following discontinuation must be weighed against the possibility that reinstatement of treatment after relapse may be associated with a poorer response.

---

**Practice points: long-term treatment...**

- Discuss long-term medication with the patient.
- Continue treatment for at least 12 months at the original effective dose level.
- If medication is to be discontinued, best done gradually over weeks and months to mitigate possible withdrawal effects, and observe for signs of relapse.

---

### 4.4.4 Somatic treatments in obsessive-compulsive disorder

Failure to respond to the above pharmacological treatments, including combination treatment with intensive inpatient and/or home-based or clinic-based therapist-assisted CBT (see Chapter 5), may indicate refractoriness to treatment. At this stage, it may be necessary to liaise with specialist services offering somatic treatments.

There is limited evidence for the efficacy of electro-convulsive therapy (ECT) in OCD (Koran et al. 2007; Lins-Martins et al. 2014; NICE 2006). Repetitive transcranial magnetic stimulation (rTMS) largely remains an experimental procedure but appears to be a promising treatment, deserving further exploration through RCTs with larger sample sizes and with greater homogeneity in clinical and demographic variables, as well as stimulation parameters and brain targets (Berlim et al. 2013). Deep brain stimulation (DBS) requires neurosurgery and also largely remains an experimental treatment at present, with evidence mainly from case series suggesting an average responder rate of around 50% (de Koning et al. 2011). To date, the main DBS targets include the anterior limb of the internal capsule, the nucleus accumbens and anterior caudate nucleus, and the anterior ventral part of the subthalamic nucleus—a nucleus embedded in the striato-pallidal circuit. The physiological mechanisms underpinning the effect of DBS remains unclear. As regards ablative neurosurgery, there are two procedures that are offered by specialist centres. Anterior cingulotomy, involving lesions placed in the dorsal ACC (Sheth et al. 2013), and anterior capsulotomy, involving lesions placed within the inferior fronto-thalamic connections within the anterior limb of the internal capsule (Ruck et al. 2003), are the commonest procedures. Both procedures are believed to modulate functioning within the cortico-striatal-thalamic circuitry. Overall, the available evidence suggests that such ablative procedures offer significant therapeutic benefits to 30–60% of patients with otherwise highly refractory OCD. There are no RCTs, and most data are derived from prospective case series and small unblinded cohort studies. Surgical intervention is therefore reserved for patients with severe, incapacitating OCD who have failed an exhaustive array of expertly delivered medication trials and intensive psychological (including behavioural) treatments. The authors recommend that readers refer to the website of the Advanced Interventions Service (Dundee, UK), for information on psychopharmacological and psychological treatments deemed 'essential' (in the UK) before proceeding to surgery.

## 4.5 Expert consensus guidelines for obsessive-compulsive disorder

Expert consensus has a role in complementing and supplementing empirical evidence. By synthesizing combined views on best practice, a broader range of pertinent clinical questions can be addressed. Moreover, such opinions reflect experience with a range of cases, and not just the highly selected groups that meet study criteria.

**Box 4.1 UK NICE guideline: key recommendations**

- Awareness of OCD as major lifespan disorder.
- Access to specialist services, according to 'stepped care model'.
- Availability of CBTs (including ERP) and pharmacotherapies (SSRIs and CMI).
- Behaviour therapy or pharmacotherapy first line for adults.
- Behaviour therapy first line, pharmacotherapy second line for children.
- Combined behaviour therapy and pharmacotherapy in more severe cases.

CBT, cognitive behavioural therapy; CMI, clomipramine; ERP, exposure and response prevention; OCD, obsessive-compulsive disorder; SSRI, selective serotonin reuptake inhibitor.

According to the Expert Consensus Panel for OCD (March et al. 1997) and the World Council on Anxiety (Greist et al. 2003), combined SRI with CBT was thought the best approach for most patients. The British Association for Psychopharmacology's (BAP) evidence-based guidelines for treating anxiety disorders, which included OCD (Baldwin et al. 2005, 2014), based its recommendations on the level of evidence adapted from the US Agency for Health Care Policy and Research Classification (US Department of Health and Human Services 1992). The BAP guideline was less certain that combination treatment was superior to psychological or serotonergic drugs given alone. NICE consulted widely over the scope of the guideline. Published and unpublished evidence supporting the efficacy of all therapies for OCD (and BDD) were subjected to a meta-analysis, wherever possible (NICE 2006). NICE emphasized the importance of better recognition of the disorder across the lifespan, and the need for good information and education. They recommended a 'stepped care' model, with increasing intensity of integrated drug and psychological treatment according to clinical severity and complexity (Box 4.1). The Canadian guidelines (Katzman et al., 2014), the American Psychiatric Association guidelines, the Cape Town consensus (Zohar et al. 2007), and the World Federation of Societies for Biological Psychiatry (Bandelow et al. 2008) guidelines are all consistent with the NICE guidelines.

For the majority of cases, this means treatment at the primary care level. For more severe or resistant cases, the guideline supported the establishment of specialist services, including national services for the most 'difficult-to-treat' individuals. NICE also paid particular attention to patient choice in directing treatment, and to the careful estimation of risks and costs of treating or not treating the disorder. For adults, either CBT or drug therapy were advocated first-line, whereas, for children, NICE considered that CBT should usually be offered before medication, because it was likely to be better tolerated, as long as appropriate CBT was readily available. Figure 4.2 summarizes guideline- based treatment options for adults with OCD.

## 4.6 **Pharmacotherapy of obsessive-compulsive and related disorders**

Compared to OCD, the evidence supporting the efficacy of pharmacotherapy in OCRDs is relatively thin. Nevertheless, SRIs do appear to be efficacious in BDD. A randomized controlled study showed efficacy for fluoxetine (40–80 mg/day), compared with placebo (Phillips et al. 2002), and another showed superiority for clomipramine over the noradrenergic antidepressant desipramine (Hollander et al. 1999). No evidence exists on the optimal dose of SSRIs in BDD, but expert opinion suggests SRIs may have a dose–response relationship akin to OCD and that the maximum tolerated dose should be tried (Ipser et al. 2009; NICE 2006). Adjunctive antipsychotic is thought to be effective in SRI-resistant cases of BDD; however, unlike OCD, this strategy has not been rigorously examined in placebo-controlled trials.

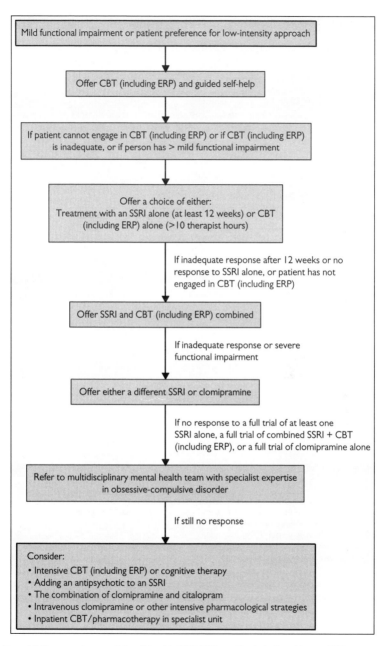

**Figure 4.2** Treatment framework for adults with OCD. CBT, cognitive behavioural therapy; ERP, exposure and response prevention; SSRI, selective serotonin reuptake inhibitor.

A single randomized trial of adjunctive pimozide was unable to detect an advantage over placebo (Phillips 2005).

Early data found that, in studies of OCD, compulsive hoarding predicted a poorer response to SSRIs (Stein *et al.* 2008). There are fewer data on the pharmacotherapy of patients who meet diagnostic criteria for hoarding disorder. Nevertheless, some studies do suggest the value of SSRIs in this condition (Saxena 2011).

Though trichotillomania may share neurocircuitry abnormalities with OCD, and some studies have reported a favourable response to SSRIs or clomipramine, the results of the treatment trials are not consistently positive. In a recent Cochrane review (Rothbart *et al.* 2013), it was concluded that none of the three eligible studies of SSRIs in trichotillomania produced strong evidence of a treatment effect, whereas the single study of clomipramine showed evidence of efficacy on several measures. Other treatments under investigation for trichotillomania include olanzapine and acetylcysteine, each of which have demonstrated a statistically significant treatment effect in a placebo-controlled study, and naltrexone.

In a review of interventions for skin-picking disorder, it was noted that the data for efficacy of SSRIs are mixed (Grant *et al.* 2012).While an open-label study of lamotrigine showed some evidence of efficacy (Grant *et al.* 2007), a follow-up double-blind placebo-controlled study failed to show any benefits (Grant *et al.* 2010).There are case reports of efficacy of opioid antagonists in skin-picking disorder (Grant *et al.* 2012). Furthermore, case reports have suggested possible benefit from riluzole (Sasso *et al.* 2006) and acetylcysteine (Odlaug *et al.* 2007) in this condition.

# References

Abramowitz JS (1997). Effectiveness of psychological and pharmacological treatments for obsessive compulsive disorder: a quantitative review. *J Consult Clin Psychol.* **65**: 44–52.

Ackerman DL and Greenland S (2002). Multivariate meta-analysis of controlled drug studies for obsessive compulsive disorder. *J Clin Psychopharmacol.* **22**: 309–17.

Aizenberg D, et al. (1999). The serotonin antagonist mianserin for treatment of serotonin-reuptake inhibitor-induced sexual dysfunction: an open-label study. *Clin Neuropharmacol.* **22**: 347–50.

Albert U, et al. (2002). Venlafaxine versus clomipramine in the treatment of obsessive–compulsive disorder: a preliminary single-blind, 12-week, controlled study. *J Clin Psychiatry.* **63**: 1004–9.

Bairy KL, et al. (2007). Developmental and behavioral consequences of prenatal fluoxetine. *Pharmacology.* **79**: 1–11.

Baldwin DS, et al. (2005). Evidence-based guidelines for the pharmacological treatment of anxiety disorders: recommendations from the British Association for Psychopharmacology. *J Psychopharmacol.* **19**: 567–96.

Baldwin DS, et al. (2014). Evidence-based pharmacological treatment of anxiety disorders, post-traumatic stress disorder and obsessive–compulsive disorder: a revision of the 2005 guidelines from the British Association for Psychopharmacology. *J Psychopharmacol.* 1–37.

Bandelow B, et al. (2008). World Federation of Societies of Biological Psychiatry (WFSBP) guidelines for the pharmacological treatment of anxiety, obsessive–compulsive and post-traumatic stress disorders: first revision. *World J Biol Psychiatry.* **9**: 248–312.

Bejerot S and Bodlund O (1998). Response to high doses of citalopram in treatment-resistant obsessive compulsive disorder. *Acta Psychopharmacol Scand.* **98**: 423–4.

Bergeron R, et al. (2001). Sertraline and fluoxetine treatment of obsessive compulsive disorder: results of a double-blind, 6-month treatment study. *J Clin Psychopharmacol.* **22**: 148–54.

Berlim MT, et al. (2013). Repetitive transcranial magnetic stimulation (r TMS) for obsessive–compulsive disorder (OCD): an exploratory meta-analysis of randomized and sham-controlled trials. *J Psychiatr Res.* **47**: 999–1006.

Berlin HA, et al. (2010). Double-blind, placebo-controlled trial of topiramate augmentation in treatment-resistant obsessive–compulsive disorder. *J Clin Psychiatry.* **72**: 716–21.

Bisserbe JC, *et al.* (1997) A double-blind comparison of sertraline and clomipramine in outpatients with obsessive–compulsive disorder. *Eur Psychiatry.* **12**: 82–93.

Bloch MH, *et al.* (2006). A systematic review: antipsychotic augmentation with treatment refractory obsessive–compulsive disorder. *Mol Psychiatry.* **11**: 622–32. Erratum in: *Mol Psychiatry.* 2006 Aug; **11**: 795.

Bloch MH, *et al.* (2010). Meta-analysis of the dose-response relationship of SSRI in obsessive–compulsive disorder. *Mol Psychiatry.* **15**: 850–5.

Bloch MH, *et al.* (2012). Effects of ketamine in treatment-refractory obsessive–compulsive disorder. *Biol Psychiatry.* **72**: 964–70.

Bogetto F, *et al.* (2002). Sertraline treatment of obsessive–compulsive disorder: efficacy and tolerability of a rapid titration regimen. *Euro Neuropsychopharmacol.* **12**: 181–6.

Bridge JA, *et al.* (2007). Clinical response and risk for reported suicidal ideation and suicide attempts in pediatric antidepressant treatment: a meta-analysis of randomized controlled trials. *J Am Med Asso.* **297**: 1683–96.

Bruno A, *et al.* (2012). Lamotrigine augmentation of serotonin reuptake inhibitors in treatment-resistant obsessive–compulsive disorder: a double-blind, placebo-controlled study. *J Psychopharmacol.* **26**: 1456–62.

Byerly MJ, *et al.* (1996). High doses of sertraline for treatment-resistant obsessive compulsive disorder. *Am J Psychiatry.* 153: 1232–3.

Bystrtitsky A, *et al.* (2004). Augmentation of serotonin re-uptake inhibitors in refractory obsessive–compulsive disorder using adjunctive olanzapine: a placebo-controlled trial. *J Clin Psychiatry.* **65**: 565–8.

Canadian Psychiatric Association (2006). Clinical practice guidelines: management of anxiety disorders. *Can J Psychiatry.* **51**, Suppl 2: 1S–92S.

Carey PD, *et al.* (2012). Quetiapine augmentation of serotonin reuptake inhibitors in treatment-refractory obsessive–compulsive disorder: is response to treatment predictable? *Int Clin Psychopharmacol.* **27**: 321–5.

Chouinard G, *et al.* (1990). Results of a double-blind placebo-controlled trial of a new serotonin re-uptake inhibitor, sertraline, in the treatment of obsessive–compulsive disorder. *Psychopharmacol Bull.* **26**: 279–84.

Clomipramine Collaborative Study Group (1991). Clomipramine in the treatment of patients with obsessive compulsive disorder. *Arch Gen Psychiatry.* **48**: 730–8.

Corá-Locatelli G, *et al.*(1998). Gabapentin augmentation for fluoxetine-treated patients with obsessive–compulsive disorder. *J Clin Psychiatry.* **59**: 480–1.

Coric V, *et al.* (2005). Riluzole augmentation in treatment-resistant obsessive–compulsive disorder: an open-label trial. *Biol Psychiatry.* **58**: 424–8.

Cottraux J, *et al.* (1990). A controlled study of fluvoxamine and exposure in obsessive–compulsive disorder. *Int Clin Psychopharmacol.* **5**: 17–30.

De Koning PP, *et al.* (2011). Current status of deep brain stimulation for obsessive–compulsive disorder: a clinical review of different targets. *Curr Psychiatry Rep.***13**: 274–82.

Denys D, *et al.* (2003). A double blind comparison of venlafaxine and paroxetine in obsessive–compulsive disorder. *J Clin Psychopharmacol.* **23**: 568–75.

Denys D, *et al.* (2004). A double-blind switch study of paroxetine and venlafaxine in obsessive–compulsive disorder. *J Clin Psychiatry.* **65**: 37–43.

De Veaugh-Geiss *et al.* (1989). Treatment of obsessive compulsive disorder with clomipramine. *Psychiat Ann.* **19**: 97–101.

De Veaugh-Geiss J, *et al.* (1992). Clomipramine hydrochloride in childhood and adolescent obsessive compulsive disorder: a multicenter trial. *J Am Acad Child Adolesc Psychiatry.* **31**: 45–9.

Diniz JB, *et al.* (2011). A double-blind, randomized, controlled trial of fluoxetine plus quetiapine or clomipramine versus fluoxetine plus placebo for obsessive–compulsive disorder. *J Clin Psychopharmacol.* **31**: 763–8.

Dold M, *et al.* (2013). Antipsychotic augmentation of serotonin reuptake inhibitors in treatment-resistant obsessive–compulsive disorder: a meta-analysis of double-blind, randomized, placebo-controlled trials. *Int J Neuropsychopharmacol.* **16**: 557–74.

Ducasse D, *et al.* (2014). D2 and D3 dopamine receptor affinity predicts effectiveness of antipsychotic drugs in obsessive–compulsive disorders: a meta regression analysis. *Psychopharmacology (Berl).* 231: 3765–70.

Fallon BA, *et al.* (1998). Intravenous clomipramine for obsessive–compulsive disorder refractory to oral clomipramine: a placebo-controlled study. *Arch Gen Psychiatry.* **55**: 918–24.

Fineberg NA and Gale T. (2005). Evidence-based pharmacological treatments for obsessive compulsive disorder. *Int J Neuropsychopharmacol.* **8**: 107–29.

Fineberg NA, et al. (1997). Brain 5-HT function in obsessive–compulsive disorder: prolactin responses to d-fenfluramine. *Br J Psychiatry*. 171: 280–2.

Fineberg N, et al. (2004). Does childhood and adult obsessive compulsive disorder (OCD) respond the same way to treatment with serotonin reuptake inhibitors (SRIs)? *Eur Neuropsychopharmacol*. **14** (Suppl. 3): S191.

Fineberg NA, et al. (2005). Adding quetiapine to SRI in treatment resistant obsessive compulsive disorder: a randomized controlled treatment study. *Int Clin Psychopharmacol*. **20**: 223–6.

Fineberg NA, et al. (2006a). Adjunctive quetiapine for SRI-resistant obsessive compulsive disorder: a meta-analysis of randomised controlled treatment trials. *Int Clin Psychopharmacol*. **21**: 337–43.

Fineberg NA, et al. (2006b). A review of antipsychotics in treatment resistant obsessive compulsive disorder (OCD). *J Psychopharmacol*. **20**: 97–103.

Fineberg N, et al. (2006c). Escitalopram in relapse prevention in patients with obsessive–compulsive disorder (OCD) *Eur Neuropsychopharmacol*. **16** (Suppl. 4): S292.

Fineberg NA, et al. (2012) Evidence-based pharmacotherapy of obsessive–compulsive disorder. *Int J Neuropsychopharmacol*. **15**: 1173–91.

Fineberg NA, et al. (2013). Pharmacotherapy of obsessive–compulsive disorder: evidence base and beyond. *Aust NZ J Psychiatry*. **47**: 121–41.

Freeman CP, et al. (1994). Fluvoxamine versus clomipramine in the treatment of obsessive–compulsive disorder: a multicenter, randomized, double-blind, parallel group comparison. *J Clin Psychiatry*. **55**: 301–5.

Geller DA, et al. (2001). Fluoxetine treatment for obsessive–compulsive disorder in children and adolescents: a placebo-controlled clinical trial *J Am Acad Child Adolesc Psychiatry*. **40**: 773–9.

Geller DA, et al. (2003a). Which SSRI? A meta-analysis of pharmacotherapy trials in paediatric obsessive–compulsive disorder. *Am J Psychiatry*. 160: 1919–28.

Geller DA, et al. (2003b). Impact of comorbidity on treatment response to paroxetine in paediatric obsessive compulsive disorder: is the use of exclusion criteria empirically supported in randomised controlled trials? *J Child Adolesc Psychopharmacol*. **13** (Suppl.): S19–29.

Geller DA, et al. (2004). Paroxetine treatment in children and adolescents with obsessive–compulsive disorder: a randomized, multicenter, double-blind, placebo-controlled trial. *J Am Acad Child Adolesc Psychiatry*. **43**: 1387–96.

Ghaliwa A, et al. (2013). Memantine add-on in moderate to severe obsessive–compulsive disorder: randomized double-blind placebo-controlled study. *J Psychiatr Res*. **47**: 175–80.

Goodman WK, et al. (1989). Efficacy of fluvoxamine in obsessive–compulsive disorder. a double-blind comparison with placebo. *Arch Gen Psychiatry*. **46**: 36–44.

Goodman WK, et al. (1996). Treatment of obsessive–compulsive disorder with fluvoxamine: a multicentre, double-blind, placebo-controlled trial. *Int. Clin. Psychopharmacol*. **11**: 21–9.

Grant JE, et al. (2007). Lamotrigine treatment of pathologic skin picking: an open label study. *J Clin Psychiatry*. **68**: 1384–91.

Grant JE, et al. (2010). A double-blind placebo-controlled trial of lamotrigine for pathological skin picking: treatment efficacy and neurocognitive predictors of response. *J Clin Psychopharmacol*. **30**; 396–403.

Grant JE, et al. (2012). Skin picking disorder. *Am J Psychiatry*. 169: 1143–9.

Greist JH, et al. (1995a). A one year double-blind placebo-controlled fixed dose study of sertraline in the treatment of obsessive–compulsive disorder. *Int Clin Psychopharmacol*. **10**: 57–65.

Grelst JH, et al. (1995b). Efficacy and tolerability of serotonin transport inhibitors in obsessive–compulsive disorder: a meta-analysis. *Arch Gen Psychiatry*. **52**: 53–60.

Greist JH, et al. (2003). Long-term treatment of obsessive–compulsive disorder in adults. *CNS Spectr*. **8**: 7–16.

Haghighi M, et al. (2013). In a double blind randomized and placebo controlled trial adjuvant memantine improved symptoms in inpatients suffering from refractory obsessive compulsive disorders OCD. *Psychopharmacology*. 228: **4**: 633–40.

Harris E, et al. (2010). Disinhibition as a side effect of treatment with fluvoxamine in pediatric patients with obsessive–compulsive disorder. *J Child Adolesc Psychopharmacol*. **20**: 347–53.

Hewlett WA, et al. (1992). Clomipramine, clonazepam, and clonidine treatment of obsessive–compulsive disorder. *J Clin Psychopharmacol*. **12**: 420–30.

Hirsch M and Birnbaum RJ (2013). Sexual dysfunction associated with selective serotonin reuptake inhibitor (SSRI) antidepressants: management. Available at: <http://www.uptodate.com/contents/

sexual-dysfunction-associated-with-selective-serotonin-reuptake-inhibitor-ssri-antidepressants-management> (accessed 5 October 2014).

Hollander E, *et al*. (1999). Clomipramine vs desipramine crossover trial in body dysmorphic disorder: selective efficacy of a serotonin reuptake inhibitor in imagined ugliness. *Arch Gen Psychiatry*. **56**: 1033–9.

Hollander E, *et al*. (2003a). A double-blind placebo-controlled study of the efficacy and safety of controlled release fluvoxamine in patients with obsessive–compulsive disorder. *J Clin Psychiatry*. **64**: 640–7.

Hollander E, *et al*. (2003b). Acute and long-term treatment and prevention of relapse of obsessive–compulsive disorder with paroxetine. *J Clin Psychiatry*. **64**: 1113–21.

Hollander E, *et al*. (2010). Quality of life outcomes in patients with obsessive–compulsive disorder: relationship to treatment response and symptom relapse. *J Clin Psychiatry*. **71**: 784–92.

Insel TR, *et al*. (1983). D-amphetamine in obsessive–compulsive disorder. *Psychopharmacology (Berl)*. **80**: 231–5.

Ipser JC, *et al*. (2006) Pharmacotherapy augmentation strategies in treatment-resistant anxiety disorders. *Cochrane Database Syst Rev*. **4**: CD005473.

Ipser JC, *et al*. (2009). Pharmacotherapy and psychotherapy for body dysmorphic disorder. *Cochrane Database Syst Rev*. **1**: CD005332.

Jenike MA, *et al*. (1990a). A controlled trial of fluvoxamine in obsessive–compulsive disorder; implications for a serotonergic theory. *Am J Psychiatry*. 147: 1209–15.

Jenike MA, *et al*. (1990b). Sertraline in obsessive–compulsive disorder: a double-blind comparison with placebo. *Am J Psychiatry*. 147: 923–8.

Jenike MA, *et al*. (1997). Placebo-controlled trial of fluoxetine and phenelzine for obsessive–compulsive disorder. *Am J Psychiatry*. 154: 1261–4.

Katzman MA, *et al*. (2014). Canadian clinical practice guidelines for the management of anxiety, posttraumatic stress and obsessive–compulsive disorders. *BMC Psychiatry*. **14** (Suppl 1).

Kobak KA, *et al*. (1998). Behavioural versus pharmacological treatments of obsessive compulsive disorder: a meta-analysis. *Psychopharmacol*. 136: 205–16.

Komossa K, *et al*. (2010). Second-generation antipsychotics for obsessive compulsive disorder. *Cochrane Database Syst Rev*. **12**: CD008141.

Koran LM and Simpson HB (2013). Guideline watch: practice guideline for the treatment of patients with obsessive–compulsive disorder. Available at: <http://psychiatryonline.org/pb/assets/raw/sitewide/practice_guidelines/guidelines/ocd-watch.pdf> (accessed 6 March 2015).

Koran LM, *et al*. (1996). Fluvoxamine versus clomipramine for obsessive–compulsive disorder: a double-blind comparison. *J Clin Psychopharmacol*. **16**: 121–9.

Koran LM, *et al*. (1997). Rapid benefit of intravenous pulse-loading of clomipramine in obsessive compulsive disorder. *Am J Psychiatry*. 154: 396–401.

Koran LM, *et al*. (2002). Efficacy of sertraline in the long-term treatment of obsessive–compulsive disorder. *Am J Psychiatry*. 159: 89–95.

Koran LM, *et al*. (2005). Mirtazapine for obsessive–compulsive disorder: an open trial followed by double-blind discontinuation. *J Clin Psychiatry*. **66**: 515–20.

Koran LM, *et al*. (2007). Practice guideline for the treatment of patients with obsessive–compulsive disorder. Arlington, VA: American Psychiatric Association. Available at: <http://psychiatryonline.org/pb/assets/raw/sitewide/practice_guidelines/guidelines/ocd.pdf> (accessed 5 March 2015).

Koran LM, *et al*. (2009). Double-blind study of dextroamphetamine versus caffeine augmentation for treatment-resistant obsessive–compulsive disorder. *J Clin Psychiatry*. **70**: 1530–5.

Kronig MH, *et al*. (1999). Placebo-controlled, multicenter study of sertraline treatment for obsessive–compulsive disorder. *J Clin Psychopharmacol*. **19**: 172–6.

Leibowitz MR, *et al*. (2002). Fluoxetine in children and adolescents with OCD: a placebo-controlled trial. *J Am Acad Child Adolesc Psychiatry*. **41**: 1431–8.

Lins-Martins NM, *et al*. (2014). Electroconvulsive therapy in obsessive–compulsive disorder: a chart review and evaluation of its potential therapeutic effects. *J Neuropsychiatry Clin Neurosci*. Aug 8. doi:10.1176/appi.neuropsych.13080184. [Epub ahead of print].

Lopez-Ibor J Jr, *et al*. (1996). Double-blind comparison of fluoxetine versus clomipramine in the treatment of obsessive–compulsive disorder. *Eur Neuropsychopharmacol*. **6**: 111–18.

Maina G, *et al*. (2003a). Weight-gain during long-term drug treatment of obsessive compulsive disorder. *Eur Neuropsychopharmacol*. **13** (Suppl.): S357.

Maina G, et al. (2003b). Antipsychotic augmentation for treatment-resistant obsessive compulsive disorder: what if antipsychotic is discontinued? Int Clin Psychopharmacol. **18**: 23–8.

March JS, et al. (1997). The Expert Consensus Guideline series. Treatment of obsessive–compulsive disorder. J Clin Psychiatry. **58** (Suppl.): 1–72.

March JS, et al. (1998). Sertraline in children and adolescents with obsessive compulsive disorder: a multicentre randomised controlled trial. J Am Med Assoc. **28**: 1752–6.

March JS, et al. (2006). Treatment benefits and the risk of suicidality in multicenter randomised controlled trials of sertraline in children and adolescents. Child Adolesc Psychopharmacol. **16**(1–2): 91–102.

Milanfranchi A, et al. (1997). A double-blind study of fluvoxamine and clomipramine in the treatment of obsessive–compulsive disorder. Int Clin Psychopharmacol. **12**: 131–6.

Monteiro WO, et al. (1987). Anorgasmia from clomipramine in obsessive–compulsive disorder: a controlled trial. Br J Psychiatry. 151: 107–112.

Montgomery SA (1980). Clomipramine in obsessional neurosis: a placebo-controlled trial. Pharmacol Med. **1**: 189–92.

Montgomery SA, et al. (1993). A double-blind placebo-controlled study of fluoxetine in patients with DSM-IIIR obsessive compulsive disorder. Eur Neuropsychopharmacol. **3**: 143–52.

Montgomery SA, et al. (2001). Citalopram 20mg, 40mg, and 60mg are all effective and well tolerated compared with placebo in obsessive–compulsive disorder. Int Clin Psychopharmacol. **16**: 75–86.

Mundo E, et al. (1997). Efficacy of fluvoxamine, paroxetine, and citalopram in the treatment of obsessive–compulsive disorder; a single-blind study. J Clin Psychopharmacol. **17**: 267–71.

National Institute for Health and Care Excellence (2006). Obsessive–compulsive disorder: core interventions in the treatment of obsessive–compulsive disorder and body dysmorphic disorder. National Collaborating Centre for Mental Health, British Psychological Society, and Royal College of Psychiatrists, UK. Available at: <http://www.nice.org.uk>.

Odlaug BL, et al. (2007). N-acetyl cysteine in the treatment of grooming disorders. J Clin Psychopharmacol. **27**: 227–9.

Oulis P, et al. (2011). Pregabalin augmentation in treatment-resistant obsessive–compulsive disorder. Int Clin Psychopharmacol. **26**: 221–4.

Pallanti S, et al. (1999). Citalopram for treatment-resistant obsessive–compulsive disorder. Eur Psychiatry. **14**: 101–6.

Pallanti S, et al. (2002). Citalopram infusions in resistant obsessive compulsive disorder: an open trial. J Clin Psychiatry. **63**: 796–801.

Pediatric OCD Treatment Study (POTS) Team (2004). Cognitive-behavior therapy, sertraline, and their combination for children and adolescents with obsessive–compulsive disorder: the Pediatric OCD Treatment Study (POTS) randomized controlled trial. JAMA. 292: 1969–76.

Perse T, et al. (1987). Fluvoxamine treatment of obsessive compulsive disorder. Am J Psychiatry. 144: 1543–8.

Phillips KA (2005). Placebo-controlled study of pimozide augmentation of fluoxetine in body dysmorphic disorder. Am J Psychiatry. 162: 377–9.

Phillips KA, et al. (2002). A randomized placebo-controlled trial of fluoxetine in body dysmorphic disorder. Arch Gen Psychiatry. **59**: 381–8.

Piccinelli M, et al. (1995). Efficacy of drug treatment in obsessive compulsive disorder. Br J Psychiatry. 166: 424–43.

Pigott TA, et al. (1990). Controlled comparisons of clomipramine and fluoxetine in the treatment of obsessive–compulsive disorder. Behavioral and biological results. Arch Gen Psychiatry. **47**: 926–32.

Rasmussen S, et al. (1997). A 2-year study of sertraline in the treatment of obsessive–compulsive disorder. Int Clin Psychopharmacol. **12**: 309–16.

Riddle MA, et al. (1992). Double-blind crossover trial of fluoxetine and placebo in children and adolescents with obsessive compulsive disorder. J Am Acad Child Adolesc Psychiatry. **31**: 1062–9.

Riddle MA, et al. (2001). Fluvoxamine for children and adolescents with obsessive compulsive disorder: a randomised, controlled multicentre trial. J Am Acad Child Adolesc Psychiatry. **40**: 222–9.

Rodriguez CI, et al. (2013). Randomized controlled crossover trial of ketamine in obsessive–compulsive disorder: proof-of-concept. Neuropsychopharmacol. **38**: 2475–83.

Romano S, et al. (2001). Long-term treatment of obsessive–compulsive disorder after an acute response: a comparison of fluoxetine versus placebo. J Clin Psychopharmacol. **21**: 46–52.

Rothbart R, et al. (2013). Pharmacotherapy for trichotillomania. Cochrane Database Syst Rev. **11**: CD007662.

Rouillon F (1998). A double-blind comparison of fluvoxamine and clomipramine in OCD. *Eur Neuropsychopharmacol*. **8** (Suppl.): 260–1.

Ruck C, *et al*. (2003). Capsulotomy for refractory anxiety disorders: long-term follow-up of 26 patients. *Am J Psychiatry*. 160: 513–21.

Sanchez C, *et al*. (2004). Escitalopram versus citalopram: the surprising role of the R-enantiomer. *Psychopharmacology (Berl)*. 174: 163–76.

Sasso DA, *et al*. (2006). Beneficial effects of the glutamate-modulating agent riluzole on disordered eating and pathological skin-picking behaviours. *J Clin Psychopharmacol*. **26**: 685–7.

Saxena S. (2011). Pharmacotherapy of compulsive hoarding. *J Clin Psychol*. **67**: 477–84.

Sheehan DV, *et al*. (1996). The measurement of disability. *Int Clin Psychopharmacol*. **11** (Suppl.): 89–95.

Sheth SA, *et al*. (2013). Limbic system surgery for treatment-refractory obsessive–compulsive disorder: a prospective long-term follow-up of 64 patients. *J Neurosurg*. 118: 491–7.

Simpson HB, *et al*. (2006). Response versus remission in obsessive compulsive disorder. *J Clin Psychiatry*. **67**: 269–76.

Smeraldi E, *et al*. (1992). Fluvoxamine versus clomipramine treatment in obsessive–compulsive disorder: a preliminary study. *New Trends Exp Clin Psychiatry*. **8**: 63–5.

Stein DJ, *et al*. (1995). Meta-analysis of pharmacotherapy trials of obsessive compulsive disorder. *Int Clin Psychopharmacol*. **10**: 11–18.

Stein DJ, *et al*. (2007). Escitalopram in obsessive–compulsive disorder: a randomized, placebo-controlled, paroxetine-referenced, fixed-dose, 24-week study. *Eur Neuropsychopharmacol*. **16** (Suppl. 4): S295.

Stein DJ, *et al*. (2008). Escitalopram in obsessive–compulsive disorder: response of symptom dimensions to pharmacotherapy. *CNS Spectr*. **13**: 492–8.

Szegedi A, *et al*. (1996). Combination treatment with clomipramine and fluvoxamine: drug monitoring, safety and tolerability data. *J Clin Psychiatry*. **57**: 257–64.

Tenney NH, *et al*. (2003). Effect of a pharmacological intervention on quality of life in patients with obsessive–compulsive disorder. *Int Clin Psychopharmacol*. **18**: 29–33.

Tollefson G, *et al*. (1994). A multicenter investigation of fixed-dose fluoxetine in the treatment of obsessive compulsive disorder. *Arch Gen Psychiatry*. **51**: 559–67.

US Department of Health and Human Services (1992). *Description of Levels of Evidence, Grades and Recommendations*. Available at: <www.pccrp.org/docs/pccrp%20section%20i.pdf> (accessed 5 March 2015).

US Food and Drug Administration (2012). *FDA Drug Safety Communication: Revised recommendations for Celexa (citalopram hydrobromide) related to a potential risk of abnormal heart rhythms with high doses*. Available at: <www.fda.gov/Drugs/DrugSafety/ucm297391.htm> (accessed 5 March 2015).

Watson HJ and Rees CS (2008). Meta-analysis of randomized controlled trials for paediatric obsessive–compulsive disorder. *J Child Psychol Psychiatry*. **49**: 489–98.

Wilens TE, *et al*. (1999). Absence of cardiovascular and adverse effects of sertraline in children and adolescents. *J Am Acad Child Adolesc Psychiatry*. **38**: 573–7.

Zivin K, *et al*. (2013). Evaluation of the FDA warning against prescribing citalopram at doses exceeding 40 mg. *Am J Psychiatry*. 170: 642–50.

Zohar J and Judge R (1996). Paroxetine versus clomipramine in the treatment of obsessive compulsive disorder. *Br J Psychiatry*. 169: 468–74.

Zohar J, *et al*. (2007). Consensus statement. *CNS Spectr*. **2** (suppl. 3): 59–63.

# Further reading

Fineberg NA, et al. (2013). Pharmacotherapy of obsessive–compulsive disorder: evidence base and beyond. *Aust NZ J Psychiatry*. **47**: 121–41.

Grant J, Odlaug BL, Chamberlain S. Clinical Guide to Obsessive Compulsive and Related Disorders. Oxford : Oxford University Press, 2014.

National Institute for Health and Care Excellence (2006) and NICE evidence update (2014) *Obsessive–compulsive disorder: core interventions in the treatment of obsessive–compulsive disorder and body dysmorphic disorder*. National Collaborating Centre for Mental Health, British Psychological Society, and Royal College of Psychiatrists, UK. Available at: <http://www.nice.org.uk>.

# Chapter 5

# Psychotherapy: an integrated approach

### Key points

- Behavioural therapy is effective in both adult and paediatric OCD.
- Exposure therapy is a key component of behavioural therapy.
- Cognitive interventions may also play a role in the treatment of OCD.
- It is useful to obtain a patient's explanatory model of their disorder.
- Both pharmacotherapy and psychotherapy reverse striatal dysfunction in OCD.

## 5.1 Introduction

In this chapter, we provide a brief introduction to the different types of psychotherapy for OCD. We then focus on the question of how to conceptualize and implement an integrated approach to the management of OCD. We do this by attempting to define the core psychobiological deficit in OCD and then considering how both pharmacotherapy and psychotherapy can reverse this dysfunction. Readers who are interested in more detail on the specific techniques employed in the CBT of OCD are referred to more specialized texts (see Chapter 7).

## 5.2 Psychotherapies for obsessive-compulsive disorder

Psychoanalytic treatment for obsessive-compulsive neurosis was described by Freud and was subsequently long thought to be an effective approach to management (Stein and Stone 1997). However, despite the contribution of psychodynamic authors to delineating the phenomenology and psychology of OCD, there is insufficient evidence to support the current use of psychoanalytic treatment for this condition (NICE 2005).

Behavioural therapy was the first psychotherapy for which careful empirical support was obtained (Marks 1997). It is useful in both adult and paediatric OCD (Greist 1994; March et al. 2001). A particularly important component of behavioural therapy appears to be exposure to the feared stimuli. The precise way in which exposure results in normalization of the CSTC circuitry remains, however, to be fully understood.

In behavioural therapy, a hierarchy of feared situations is created, and the patient then practises facing the fear (exposure), while monitoring the anxiety and experiencing that it lessens without the need to carry out a neutralizing ritual (response prevention). It is thought that the repeated experience of fear extinction in the context of prolonged exposure to the fear-inducing stimulus is critical to the therapeutic effect. Many individuals with OCD engage in covert mental rituals or reassurance seeking as a way of attempting to control their anxiety (Purdon 2008). These symptoms are also amenable to exposure and response prevention (ERP), which needs to be carefully crafted to the individual's behavioural repertoire. It is crucial to begin by educating the patient about the way in which the therapy works, so that they understand the importance of the exposure exercises, and to then engage the patient by using a graded programme and collaboratively tackling the easiest challenges first. Homework practice is also a crucial part of the therapy.

There may also be a role for cognitive interventions in the treatment of OCD (Salkovskis 1999). Several belief domains are likely to be important in OCD, including inflated responsibility, overimportance of thoughts, excessive concern about the importance of controlling one's thoughts, and overestimation of threat (Obsessive Compulsive Cognitions Working Group 1997; Tolin DF et al. 2006). These kinds of faulty reasoning are able to serve as targets in the cognitive therapy.

Cognitive approaches encourage patients to re-evaluate overvalued beliefs, to regain a more realistic perspective on the importance of their thoughts, and to carry out 'behavioural experiments' to test the validity of their beliefs about control and threat. Cognitive approaches may be as effective as exposure procedures, but it is not clear whether the addition of cognitive techniques significantly improves the efficacy of ERP (Abramowitz 1997; NICE 2005; van Balkom et al. 1994). Prior treatment with cognitive therapy may be especially helpful in improving treatment readiness and adherence to ERP (Sookman et al. 2003).

In practice, given that ERP may require some change in cognition prior to its use, there is an overlap between these approaches, and, in clinical settings, a 'cognitive behavioural' approach is often used, administered individually or in groups, with the contexts ranging from self-help computer instruction through to intensive hospitalization (Bachofen et al. 1999; Thornicroft et al. 1991). Given that there may be significant family accommodation to OCD symptoms, which may be associated with a poorer clinical outcome, assessing such accommodation and including the patient's partner or family in developing a treatment strategy is appropriate in some cases, particularly children and adolescents with OCD (Calvocoressi et al. 1999; Pinto et al. 2013). A recent large study showed that family-based CBT, including strategies to overcome family accommodation, is an effective treatment in children as young as 5 years of age (Freeman et al. 2014).

### 5.2.1 Overcoming potential obstacles to cognitive behavioural therapy in obsessive-compulsive disorder

It is apparent that up to 50% of those with OCD do not benefit from CBT. Avoidance and safety-seeking behaviours are very common in those suffering from OCD (Helbig-Lang and Peterman 2010), and this feature may interfere with exposure (Abramowitz et al. 2003). Other factors that may adversely affect treatment outcome include high levels of disgust, intrusive imagery (de Houwer et al. 2001), and perfectionism (Pinto et al. 2011). Severe depression has also been shown to be a poor prognostic indicator for CBT outcome (Abramowitz et al. 2007; Keeley et al. 2008), although not necessarily for pharmacological treatment (Mawson et al. 1982; Zitterl et al. 2000). Individuals with ego-syntonic obsessive symptoms or overvalued ideas may also struggle to achieve success with ERP (Neziroglu et al. 2004)

Cognitive strategies have been designed to address many of these obstacles, although further work is needed to determine their efficacy (Whittal et al. 2005). Cognitive therapy may also target complex symptoms that interfere with exposure. These include a sense of incompleteness (Summerfeldt 2004), intolerance of distress, memory confidence (Radomsky et al. 2010), risk aversion (Sookman and Steketee 2007), and metacognitive processing related to basic experience of self and world (Wells 2011). These cognitive errors are hypothesized to impact the appraisal of cognitive and emotional events.

To be successful, CBT for OCD also depends upon a supportive, collaborative, and well-defined therapeutic relationship, which emphasizes the patients' willingness to make changes. One possible obstacle is that the interpersonal dysfunction associated with OCD cognitions, e.g. manifested as an overwhelming need to be in control of thoughts and actions, may substantially interfere with the collaborative relationship between the therapist and the patient and hamper the working alliance. Alternatively, the cognitive rigidity associated with OCD, manifested, for example, as attentional set-shift problems on laboratory-based neurocognitive tasks (Chamberlain et al. 2005), may actively impede the ability to effect enduring adaptive behavioural changes. Therefore, clinicians and researchers continue to examine alternative forms of psychological treatment for this large clinical population.

In recent years, there has been a shift toward strategies that promote the acceptance of symptoms and traits. The acceptance and commitment therapy (ACT) treatment model consists of awareness and non-judgemental acceptance of all experiences, both positive and negative, identification of valued life directions, and appropriate action toward goals that support those values. Patients are encouraged to invest energy in committed actions, such as actively engaging in leisure, social, or occupational activities, rather than struggle against psychological events. Other 'third wave' CBTs, such as mindfulness therapy, are also under investigation in pilot studies. These strategies are simple to apply and review in the outpatient clinic and, although not so far rigorously tested in OCD trials, in the authors' experience, are likely to have practical value for this patient group.

Developed for eating disorder, cognitive remediation therapy (CRT) targets attention to detail and set-shifting, encourages flexible behaviour, and increases motivation and perceived ability to change. Two small-scale trials in OCD, employing approaches similar to CRT, were effective in improving obsessive-compulsive symptoms, as well as executive skills and cognitive flexibility, respectively (Buhlmann et al. 2006; Park et al. 2006). In eating disorder, CRT was shown to improve quality of life and dropout rates when combined with treatment as usual. Interestingly, cognitive inflexibility predicted a better response to CRT (Dingemans et al. 2014). CRT may thus be a beneficial adjunct to CBT in disorders characterized by cognitive inflexibility such as OCD.

From a theoretical viewpoint, there may be value in integrating different treatment modalities (Stein et al. 2001), and increasing evidence supports the use of adjunctive pharmacotherapy with SSRIs in combination with CBT to improve outcomes (Cuijpers et al. 2014). There is relatively little empirical data addressing the question of how best to sequence pharmacotherapy and psychotherapy for OCD (see Section 5.8). In clinical practice, it would seem sensible to encourage patients who are on medication also to understand and adhere to the principles of CBT, and a number of studies support the value of adding a CBT intervention to OCD patients on medication. For example, a recent randomized controlled study (Simpson et al. 2013) found that the addition of adjunctive CBT to SSRI in patients who had only made a partial response to SSRI monotherapy produced a significant further improvement both in the short term and after 6 months' follow-up (Foa et al. 2013).

## 5.3 What is the core psychobiological deficit in obsessive-compulsive disorder?

An integrated approach to the treatment of OCD would ideally rest on the basis of a clear understanding of the nature of the core psychobiological deficit underlying the disorder. Despite significant neurobiological advances in the field, defining a core psychobiological deficit in OCD remains an ambitious undertaking. As a first step toward this goal, we would tentatively suggest that the fundamental deficiency in OCD revolves around faults in the selection, maintenance, and termination of 'procedural strategies', particularly (but not exclusively) those involving harm assessment.

This characterization requires some explanation. We can begin by recalling that the bulk of current evidence—neuropsychological, neuroimaging, neuroimmunological, and neurosurgical—emphasizes the role of CSTC dysfunction in OCD (de Vries et al. 2014; Fineberg et al. 2010; Whiteside et al. 2004). The immediate question then is what the normal role of these circuits is. From there, it might be possible to determine the nature of the core dysfunction in OCD.

It is widely believed that CTSC circuits play a role in organizing motor and cognitive procedural strategies (Fineberg et al. 2014). Take, for example, the procedure for riding a bicycle. When we initially learn to ride, the effort requires a good deal of conscious concentration, involving cortical structures. However, over time, the brain–mind encodes a 'bicycling procedure'—this procedure is enacted non-consciously and automatically under the direction of the striatum. Even when we lose our explicit memories of learning to ride a bicycle, our implicit knowledge of how to ride remains (this kind of dissociation has been documented, e.g. in studies of dementia).

There is evidence suggesting that the neural mechanisms underlying procedural knowledge are disrupted in OCD. Rigorous studies of cognitive inflexibility (Chamberlain et al. 2008) and of habitual responses (Gillan et al. 2014) have contributed to our understanding of these disruptions (see further text in this section). For example, when undertaking an implicit cognition task during functional brain imaging, normal controls demonstrated the activation of CSTC circuits (especially striatal), but OCD patients showed a pathological activation of temporal regions instead (Rauch et al. 1997). Of course, OCD is not a dysfunction in bicycling; rather, OCD typically involves those procedures that involve the assessment of harm and the selection, initiation, maintenance, and termination of appropriate remediative acts, which may require consideration of more complex neuropsychological concepts, such as 'impulsivity' and 'compulsivity', and their related neuroanatomy. Moreover, results of functional neuroimaging studies in OCD have generally noted increased activation of limbic and ventral frontal-striatal regions at rest, and decreased responsiveness of dorsal frontal-striatal regions during executive performance, thus suggesting an imbalance between the dorsal and ventral striatum as the possible reason for the disruption in the CSTC circuits (van den Heuvel et al. 2005).

Impulsivity may be defined as 'a predisposition toward rapid, unplanned reactions to internal (thoughts or feelings) or external (events) stimuli with diminished regard to the negative consequences of these reactions to the impulsive individual or to others' (Chamberlain and Sahakian 2007; Potenza 2007). In contrast, compulsivity may be viewed as a tendency to perform unpleasantly repetitive acts in a habitual or stereotyped manner to prevent perceived negative consequences, leading to functional impairment (Chamberlain et al. 2006; Fineberg et al. 2010). These two constructs may be viewed as diametrically opposed, or alternatively as similar, in that each implies a dysfunction of impulse control (Stein and Hollander 1993a). Each potentially involves alteration within a wide range of neural processes, including attention, perception, and coordination of motor or cognitive responses.

In a series of laboratory-based studies, patients with OCD and their unaffected first-degree relatives were found to show abnormally high levels of 'motor impulsivity' on neurocognitive tasks. This was manifested as a relative failure to inhibit motor responses, once they had been generated. It may represent a neuropsychological correlate of the failure to inhibit OCD compulsions once they have been initiated. Moreover, structural abnormalities were seen in grey and white matter areas of the brain that correlated with the severity of the motor deficit (Menzies et al. 2007). In another series of experiments, patients and their unaffected relatives were found to underactivate the OFC when performing a task that requires reversal learning—a process whereby individuals learn to switch away from responses that are no longer rewarding (Chamberlain et al. 2008). In yet further work, OCD patients and their unaffected relatives showed problems in flexibly shifting attention from one task to another, reflecting the 'cognitive rigidity' observed in OCD whereby patients focus their attention and behavioural responses on specific ideas and actions without being able to flexibly move on (Chamberlain et al. 2007a) These family-based deficits suggest the existence of brain-based primary processing problems that interfere with stopping and switching away from unrewarding motor behaviours as a vulnerability factor for compulsivity in OCD.

There is growing interest in the overlap between the neurobiology of OCD and of more impulsive conditions, including the addictions. Neuroanatomical models posit the existence of separate, but intercommunicating, 'compulsive' and 'impulsive' cortico-striatal circuits, differentially modulated by neurotransmitters (Fineberg et al. 2010) that are each likely to contribute to the generation of OCD symptoms such as intrusive, unwanted thoughts and behaviours. In the compulsive circuit, a striatal component (caudate nucleus) may drive compulsive behaviours, and a prefrontal component (OFC) may exert inhibitory control over them. Similarly, in the impulsive circuit, a striatal component (ventral striatum/nucleus accumbens shell) may drive impulsive behaviours, and a prefrontal component (ACC/VMPFC) may exert inhibitory control. Other important areas for cortical control include the lateral prefrontal cortex (PFC), especially on the right side, and increasingly (but mainly in social cognition or reward-based choice procedures) the dorsolateral PFC. Thus, in this OCD model, there exist at least two striatal neural circuitries (one compulsive and one impulsive) that drive OCD-related behaviours, and two corresponding prefrontal circuitries that restrain them. Hyperactivity within the striatal components or abnormalities (presumably hypoactivity) in the prefrontal components may thus result in an increased automatic tendency for executing impulsive or compulsive behaviours, depending on the sub-component affected.

Other neuroanatomical models emphasize a cognitive–affective diathesis that may explain the link between OCD and harm-related thoughts and activities. Such models propose that, within the fronto-striatal circuitry, there may be over-activation of ventral components, including OFC, that may drive the 'urge' to perform an OCD-related behaviour, and under-activation of dorsal components, including the ACC (Vriend et al. 2013) and dorsal frontal cortex (de Vries et al. 2014), that normally exert executive control over behavioural responses to allow the appropriate selection, initiation, timing, stopping, etc. of purposeful acts that is also essential for effective planning and problem-solving. Indeed, patients with OCD are noted to be poor at executive planning on laboratory-based tasks and to show an abnormal attentional bias connected to negatively valenced emotional stimuli such as sad faces (Chamberlain et al. 2007b). Some of the authors suggest that neural inefficiency within the dorsal fronto-parietal network during task performance contributes to compulsive activity, and furthermore that the disruption may result from limbic interference such as from increased activation of the amygdala fear circuitry (de Vries et al. 2014). Thus, abnormal fear processing may directly impact on OCD-related neurocircuitry to generate specific alterations in cognitive–affective processes, such as exaggerated harm assessment, and alterations in emotions, such as disgust, leading onward to the generation of obsessions and compulsions (Milad and Rauch 2012).

The fact that areas of the OFC, rather than the amygdala, are predominantly activated in brain imaging studies of OCD suggests that the stimuli which generate anxiety for the OCD sufferer originate internally, rather than externally. Similarly, work emphasizing the role of disgust and the insula cortex in OCD and some anxiety disorders emphasizes the role of interoceptive processes. Data suggest that the insula is important in coordinating 'conscious' urges. Exposure to cues in the environment, or homeostatic states such as withdrawal, stress, disgust, or anxiety, may evoke 'interoceptive' representations in the insula that translate into consciously perceived 'urges'. The insula is anatomically and functionally connected to the cortico-striatal neural systems implicated in impulsivity, compulsivity, and inhibitory control. Conceivably, the insula interacts with mechanisms of impulsivity and compulsivity by relaying signals (from the environment or the viscera) to the PFC. Thus, interoceptive signals mediated through the insula may, on the one hand, sensitize the neural circuits driving impulsivity or compulsivity. On the other hand, insula activity may 'hijack' the inhibitory control mechanisms of the PFC and subvert attention, reasoning, planning, and decision-making processes away from foreseeing the negative consequences of a given action, and toward formulating plans to execute it (Naqvi et al. 2007). It could be hypothesized that, in OCD, once a trigger—say a speck of dirt—has been noticed, an internal cognitive process, perhaps comprising exaggerated insula activity, disrupts the cortico-striatal processing, resulting in the exaggeration of its potential harmful consequences and generating compulsive activity designed to reduce anxiety and disgust.

However, an important series of experiments, during which patients with OCD learn to avoid a potentially harmful stimulus, has challenged the traditional notion that obsessions relating to an exaggerated fear of harm drive OCD. In these studies, compared to healthy controls, OCD patients demonstrated changes in OFC activation that were accompanied by excessive habitual (stimulus-dependent) avoidance responses that persevered, even when the potentially harmful stimulus was no longer present. Moreover, repetition of the avoidance habits appeared to generate new, never previously experienced, harm-related 'obsessional' fears that were related specifically to the experimental procedure, as a means of justifying the excessive avoidance behaviour. This fascinating finding, i.e. that, in OCD patients, the habitual repetition of avoidance behaviours unrelated to their OCD can generate de novo rationalizations in the form of new harm-related fears, suggests that habit mechanisms: (a) contribute to the development of motor compulsions and (b) may additionally act to generate harm-related obsessional thoughts, rather than vice versa (Gillan et al. 2013).

## 5.4 Core deficit versus compensatory dysfunctions

One of the interesting challenges in interpreting the neuroimaging literature in OCD is the fact that many functional imaging studies report over-activation in areas of the OFC. Such studies have tended to focus on resting state or symptom provocation paradigms, and the area of overactivity appears to be focused around the medial aspects of the OFC (Saxena and Rauch 2000). However, other studies, such as those investigating 'neutral' task performance such as reversal learning, demonstrated underactivation of the OFC, predominantly in lateral areas (Chamberlain et al. 2008). These apparently conflicting findings could be explained by the existence of functional subdivisions within the OFC, with some areas showing overactivity (medial), and others underactivity (lateral), during different forms of cognitive processing.

Although it is possible that increased medial orbitofrontal activation represents a primary lesion in OCD, it is also possible that this is instead a compensatory response. In this view, orbitofrontal activation represents a compensatory reaction to dysfunction in subcortical structures, along the lines of a 'natural defence' against obsessional anxiety. Thus, increased activity in selected areas within the OFC may represent an attempt to suppress striatally mediated harm exaggeration in OCD. It has been suggested that one of the roles of treatment may be to bolster this 'natural defence' mechanism.

The finding that OCD patients with low orbitofrontal activity on brain imaging prior to treatment are less likely to respond to medication (Swedo et al. 1992) is in line with this hypothesis. It is as if there is not enough capacity in the system for adequate compensation to be achieved. Similarly, it is interesting that the behavioural exacerbation of OCD by sumatriptan, a specific agonist of the terminal autoreceptor (5-HT$_{1D}$), appears to be associated with decreased activity in areas of the PFC (Stein et al. 1999), perhaps suggesting that the level of activity in the compensatory circuitry has been turned down by the drug.

It is notable that certain serotonergic systems appear underactive in untreated OCD (e.g. blunted prolactin response to the serotonergic agonist mCPP) (Hollander *et al.* 1992; Zohar *et al.* 1987), as well as in impulsivity (Stein and Hollander 1993a). The cognitive process whereby a speck of dirt triggers exaggerated fear of harm (by contamination) and sets off handwashing compulsions may well reflect striatal serotonergic hypofunction. Conversely, there is also evidence of hyperserotonergic function in OCD (e.g. enhanced growth hormone responses to L-tryptophan and dexfenfluramine) (Fineberg *et al.* 1994, 1997) and symptom exacerbation after mCPP (Hollander *et al.* 1992; Zohar *et al.* 1987), and this may represent prefrontal compensatory mechanisms at work.

This view of underlying deficit and secondary compensation in OCD provides a speculative way of tying together a range of neuroanatomical and neurochemical findings. But does it make sense in terms of our clinical understanding of the symptomatology and experience of suffering from OCD?

One of the most convincing descriptions of the phenomenology of OCD turns out to be that of Freud. Indeed, Freud's understanding of obsessional neurosis provides a cornerstone for psychodynamic theory and is consistent with much modern thinking about the operation of an unconscious. For Freud, at the heart of obsessional neurosis are unconscious aggressive instincts (Freud 1926). Unacceptable urges, particularly hostile urges, are admitted into awareness, because of incomplete repression, necessitating defensive responses, in the form of compulsive rituals, to reduce guilt and anxiety.

This formulation is redolent of the psychobiological characterization already described. In OCD, there may be a non-conscious, striatally mediated impulsive/disinhibited process. This results in frontally mediated compensatory attempts to switch this process off. A range of more recent data support a link between OCD and behavioural disinhibition. Epidemiological data indicate that OCD is frequently associated with a history of childhood impulsivity and aggression (Hollander and Cohen 1996). Furthermore, in clinical settings, individuals with OCD often demonstrate a degree of impulsive aggression (Stein and Hollander 1993b), which, given their harm avoidance, is counterintuitively high. Reviewing the evidence to date, it is clear that further work is needed to determine which cognitive deficits in OCD are core and which are better understood as compensatory.

## 5.5 **Doubt and uncertainty in obsessive-compulsive disorder**

So far, we have concentrated on the central theme of harm assessment and avoidance in OCD. Other authors (e.g. Tallis 1995) have drawn attention to the role of doubt in this disorder. According to Freud, doubt leads the patient to uncertainty about his protective measures and to his continual repetition of them in order to banish that uncertainty. It is as though obsessional patients have lost the ability to register they have done something or even to 'know if they know something' (Rapoport 1989).

Summerfeldt (2004) proposed the existence of two core dimensions in OCD, 'incompleteness' and 'harm avoidance,' that each has unique affective, cognitive, and motivational characteristics. Incompleteness, representing an inner sense of imperfection or the uncomfortable subjective state that one's actions or experiences are not 'just right,' was proposed as a temperament-like motivational variable within OCD that results in symmetry, counting, repeating and slowness. A sense of incompleteness also characterizes obsessive-compulsive personality disorder. Indeed, high incompleteness scores in patients with OCD are predictive of meeting criteria for comorbid obsessive-compulsive personality disorder, suggesting the presence of the comorbid disorder exerts a pathoplastic effect on the OCD (Summerfeldt *et al.* 2004).

It has been suggested that dysfunction of CSTC circuits may interfere with the normal verification of the successful completion of preventive or reparative behaviours, leading to compulsive repetition of the behaviours until appropriate information processing is accomplished (Stein and Hollander 1993; Zor et al. 2011). Alternatively, a sense of heightened personal responsibility and/or need for a perfect outcome could drive the need to perform tasks with absolute certainty and generate anxiety, doubt, and the need to check. In a recent study, using video-telemetry, the authors explored these alternative hypotheses by documenting the behavioural manifestation of incompleteness in patients enacting their usual compulsive rituals, predicting that an exaggerated focus on 'functional' acts appropriate for the motor task would support the hypothesis that heightened responsibility/perfectionism was the driver. In contrast, increased 'non-functional' activity occurring after the expected terminal act for the task would support the 'stop signal deficiency' hypothesis. The results showed high rates of non-functional activity occurring predominantly after the functional end of the activity, supporting the 'lack of stop signal' theories as the underlying mechanism in OCD (Zor et al. 2011). Just how the compulsion eventually stops is not clear; perhaps the energy dissipates, a little like that of a tuning fork.

## 5.6 Does neurocognitive dysfunction influence treatment response in obsessive-compulsive disorder?

There is mixed evidence with regard to the prognostic role of neurocognitive functions for treatment response. A study of 138 OCD patients indicated that most neurocognitive measures did not predict treatment response, although trends in the direction of poorer outcome were found for several measures relating to cognitive flexibility such as performance on an alternation test and perseveration errors on the Wisconsin card sort test (Moritz et al. 2005). A study of 63 paediatric OCD patients indicated that, on a broader level, diminished memory and executive functions may have a negative effect on treatment response to CBT in children with OCD (Flessner et al. 2010).

## 5.7 An integrated approach to treatment

If the core psychobiological dysfunction in OCD revolves around fronto-striatally mediated problems in the selection, maintenance, and termination of procedural strategies, how might we approach treatment?

First, serotonergic medication can be used to optimize fronto-striatal function, either by direct actions at receptors in the striatum or by augmenting orbito-striatal compensatory mechanisms, as described previously. Where striatal damage is more extensive, dopamine blockers may provide an additional mechanism for increased serotonergic neuronal activity, since dopaminergic neurons act to inhibit striatal serotonergic neurons (Fineberg and Gale 2005; McDougle et al. 2000). Glutamate is a ubiquitous neurotransmitter in the CSTC circuitry and is thought to be particularly important, together with dopamine and acetylcholine, in the regulation of neuronal plasticity and habit learning in the dorsal striatum (Lovinger 2010). There is growing interest in the role of glutamatergic agents in OCD, with recent positive findings in small RCTs of ketamine and memantine; these agents may also have a role in targeting alterations in the fronto-striatal circuitry.

Second, cognitive behavioural techniques can be used to regulate fronto-striatal function. Imaging studies indicate that exposure to feared stimuli ultimately also results in optimization of the CTSC circuits. Baxter's elegant work, showing comparable effects of an SSRI and behavioural therapy on the functional neuroanatomy of OCD, remains a key support for the idea of an integrated brain–mind approach to OCD (Baxter et al. 1992). Subsequent studies have consolidated and expanded this early work (Benazon et al. 2003; Porto et al. 2009).

Third, there may be a range of preventative interventions that can be applied early in life to protect the striatum. The basal ganglia are particularly vulnerable to neonatal hypoxaemia, and preventing this is therefore important. The finding that childhood emotional deprivation is associated with neuroanatomical abnormalities in the striatum (Martin et al. 1991) provides an even more challenging area for therapeutic intervention.

Finally, autoimmune processes in the aftermath of infection with Streptococcus may also result in striatal damage. It is proposed that antibodies raised against streptococcal proteins cross-react with neuronal proteins (antigens) in the brain, particularly in the basal ganglia, which is a brain region implicated in OCD pathogenesis (Swedo et al. 1998). Hypotheses related to the existence of PANDAS as a well-defined, isolated clinical entity focused around childhood tic and obsessive-compulsive symptomatology and underpinned by definite pathophysiological mechanism (Swedo and Grant 2005) have not been convincingly supported by research evidence. In particular, the core feature represented by the association between newly diagnosed infections and neuropsychiatric symptom relapses in youths with this diagnosis could not be demonstrated by longitudinal studies. Given the uncertainties on the clinical definition of PANDAS, it is not surprising that evidence in support of a post-infectious immune-mediated pathophysiology is also insufficient. Moreover, evidence in favour of the efficacy of antibiotic prophylaxis or tonsillectomy in patients fulfilling Swedo's criteria for PANDAS is lacking, whereas a response to immune-mediated treatments, like intravenous immunoglobulins, has been documented by one study but needs replication in larger trials (Macerollo and Martino 2013). However, the finding of increased levels of anti-basal ganglia antibodies in adults, as well as children, with OCD supports the hypothesis that central nervous system autoimmunity may have an aetiological role in some individuals with OCD. Further study is required to examine whether the antibodies concerned are pathogenic and whether exposure to streptococcal infection in vulnerable individuals is a risk factor for the development of OCD (Nicholson et al. 2012).

## 5.8 Are integrated treatments more effective in obsessive-compulsive disorder?

We know that SRIs and behaviour therapy are individually effective in OCD, and it would therefore seem likely that the combination of both treatments would provide even better efficacy. In fact, there have been few studies looking at this area (NICE 2005). Meta-analyses (e.g. Cuijpers et al. 2014) have not fully succeeded in addressing the question of relative efficacy of interventions, partly because this kind of statistical approach cannot adequately correct for the changes that have occurred between individual trials over the years (e.g. rising placebo–response rates over the past 10 years, greater numbers of treatment-resistant and atypical patients entering later medication trials; see Chapter 4). However, the existing data suggest that combined treatment appears to be more effective than treatment with SSRI medication alone. These effects remain strong and significant up to 2 years after treatment (Cuijpers et al. 2014). Head-to-head comparisons of the effects of combination treatment compared with drug or behavioural monotherapy are preferable, and it is regrettable that so few properly controlled studies have been performed.

Early influential studies by Marks et al. (1980, 1988) were the first to address the question of how best to sequence and combine pharmacotherapy and psychotherapy in OCD. Their first study suggested that the addition of clomipramine to behaviour therapy enhanced compliance and produced a more favourable outcome (Marks et al. 1980). These results were echoed in the second study where the addition of clomipramine to exposure therapy produced a greater level of improvement (Marks *et al.* 1988). Unfortunately, these studies are limited by a number of methodological problems, including the use of rather small sample sizes.

Two small studies (Cottraux *et al.* 1990; Hohagen *et al.* 1998) compared fluvoxamine plus behaviour therapy with placebo plus behaviour therapy and, in spite of small numbers, demonstrated superior efficacy for the combination over exposure monotherapy for up to 6 months. There was no drug monotherapy arm in one of the studies (Hohagen *et al.* 1998). The study by Cottraux *et al.* (1990) was unable to show a significant advantage for combined drug and exposure, compared with fluvoxamine, even though the drug was given in combination with anti-exposure instructions (which should have had an adverse effect), but the study was probably underpowered (*n* = 40), and the authors themselves advocated further larger studies. A trial undertaken with a larger sample of children and adolescents with OCD found that sertraline alone, CBT alone, and CBT plus sertraline were all better than placebo, but they did not differ significantly from one another (March *et al.* 2006).

However, two recent trials have demonstrated benefit from combining pharmacotherapy with psychotherapy. An 8-week RCT in non-/partial responders to SSRI compared the augmentation of SRI treatment with 17 sessions of CBT to a matched number of sessions of stress management training and found a clear advantage for CBT in reducing Y-BOCS scores (Simpson *et al.* 2008). Another recent study, conducted by the same group in a similar patient sample, showed that augmenting SSRI with CBT was superior to adjunctive risperidone or pill placebo (Simpson *et al.* 2013). Optimistic claims from inadequately controlled studies that CBT prevents relapse if medication is prematurely discontinued (e.g. Biondi *et al.* 2005; March *et al.* 1994; Simpson *et al.* 2004), although intuitively persuasive, need to be explored further under properly controlled conditions.

## 5.9 An integrated approach in practice

So far, this chapter has been rather theoretical. How does an integrated approach work in practice?

The first step of treatment is a comprehensive psychiatric and medical history and examination. Particular symptoms in OCD (such as tics) and comorbid disorders (such as depression) may well influence the choice of intervention. Evaluation of OCD symptoms with a scale, such as the Y-BOCS (see Appendices), is useful in determining treatment targets. During these initial interactions with the patient, conveying an empathic appreciation of the experience of OCD is crucial for strengthening the clinician–patient relationship, and this kind of effect may even have contributed to the efficacy of placebo in recent clinical trials. Patients are often relieved to realize from the direction of the clinicians' questions that other patients also suffer from intensely embarrassing symptoms (such as intrusive sexual obsessions).

Once the patient has been appropriately evaluated and diagnosed, it is important to begin a process of psycho-education. In many ways, this is the first step of CBT. It is important to begin by asking the patient for their 'explanatory model' of OCD—what are their ideas about the cause of their symptoms (Stein and Rapoport 1996)? Often people misconstrue symptoms as reflecting unconscious guilt or as pointing toward a hidden personality fault. The shame that is associated with the experience of OCD (e.g. feeling incompetent for being unable to control an ego-dystonic compulsion) is presumably one of the reasons for the long lag-time between the start of OCD symptoms and seeking treatment (Hollander *et al.* 1997). The clinician can present an alternative view of OCD as a fronto-striatal 'false alarm' (as outlined in different words in earlier text) and then negotiate with the patient to try to achieve a shared understanding and treatment plan.

The question of psycho-education raises the role of consumer advocacy; this would seem increasingly relevant to an integrated approach to the treatment of OCD. Modern media allow for rapid communication of ideas and for bringing together clinicians and consumers electronically. Internet-based CBT could save the therapist time, compared to traditional treatment. It has the potential to be a cost-effective alternative in treating OCD and may improve treatment accessibility (Grifffiths *et al*. 2006). Stigmatization of mental illness can be addressed by providing appropriate information, referral to support groups, etc. Virtual support groups can also be immensely useful for people with OCD (Stein 1997).

Apps have been introduced that can be downloaded to one's phone. 'OCFighter™' (<http://www.ocfighter.com/>) and 'OCD Manager' (<http://ocd4iphone.wordpress.com/>) are two such apps that are tools that could assist the sufferer with ERP and CBT. Given the early onset of OCD symptoms, there would seem to be a need for future targeting of information about OCD and other psychiatric disorders to youngsters and to the professions (e.g. teaching) that are most often in contact with this population.

Once treatment itself begins, either medication or CBT can be chosen, depending on a range of factors, including symptom severity, comorbid illness (e.g. depression), and patient choice. (We use the term 'CBT', as cognitive interventions may also have a role in the treatment of OCD, although the majority of evidence for the efficacy of psychotherapy in OCD has focused on the value of exposure per se). Despite the relatively limited database discussed earlier, most clinicians conservatively advocate combined pharmacotherapy and psychotherapy, if available, in a stepped-care way (see Chapter 4). If medication is to be discontinued, it would seem wise to do this gradually over a period of months and to stress again the principles of exposure therapy during this time.

Drug treatment is generally available and can be monitored by a primary care practitioner, except where unusually high doses of medication or augmentation strategies are employed. CBT for OCD is generally less accessible and usually requires referral to a specialist centre where there are often long waiting lists for treatment. However, the psychotherapy component of exposure therapy is not difficult to learn and can be taught to a range of mental health professionals. Indeed, there would seem to be a demand from community psychiatric nurses to learn these skills.

Next, it is useful to incorporate the family and 'significant others' into the treatment plan. It is important, for example, to assess the adverse effects of the patient's symptoms on family function (Freeman *et al*. 2014). Furthermore, behavioural techniques may not be effective when the family works (sometimes in good faith) to prevent exposure. For example, when a patient with contamination concerns has an equally fastidious spouse, there is often mutual reinforcement to exclude exposure, and the couple must therefore be treated as a whole.

### 5.9.1 Hospitalization

In refractory patients, partial or full hospitalization (Boschen *et al*. 2008) may be a useful option for ensuring that both optimal pharmacotherapy and psychotherapy are given. Referral to a specialist unit for OCD, where both modalities of treatment (as well as expertise in neurosurgery) are available, should be considered in patients who have failed initial pharmacotherapy, psychotherapy, or combined treatments. Fortunately, however, the majority of people with OCD can be treated on an outpatient basis and will respond to simple combinations of psycho-education, an SRI, and exposure therapy.

## 5.10 Conclusion

Although much remains to be understood about the neurobiology of OCD, there is a convergence on certain hypotheses, and fronto-striatal dysfunction, in particular, appears key. Remarkably, both psychotherapy and pharmacotherapy result in the normalization of fronto-striatal function. Taken together, this means that OCD provides an extraordinarily powerful model of a contemporary approach to the brain–mind, to psychopathology, and to treatment. In the clinical setting, it is useful to be able to educate the patient that the 'false alarm' in their brain–mind can be reset through a combination of pharmacotherapy and ERP therapy. For researchers, determining the precise mechanisms through which these interventions operate remains an exciting challenge for the future.

# References

Abramowitz JS (1997). Effectiveness of psychological and pharmacological treatments for obsessive–compulsive disorder: a quantitative review. *J Consult Clin Psychol*. **65**: 44–52.

Abramowitz JS, et al. (2003). Symptom presentation and outcome of cognitive-behavioral therapy for obsessive–compulsive disorder. *J Consult Clin Psychol*. **71**: 1049–57.

Abramowitz JS, et al. (2007). Obsessive–compulsive disorder with comorbid major depressive disorder: what is the role of cognitive factors? *Behav Res Ther*. **45**: 2257–67.

Bachofen M, et al. (1999). Home self-assessment and self-treatment of obsessive–compulsive disorder using a manual and a computer-conducted telephone interview: replication of a UK–US study. *J Clin Psychiatry*. **60**: 545–9.

Baxter LR, et al. (1992). Caudate glucose metabolic rate changes with both drug and behaviour therapy for OCD. *Arch Gen Psychiatry*. **49**: 681–9.

Benazon NR, et al. (2003). Neurochemical analyses in pediatric obsessive–compulsive disorder in patients treated with cognitive-behavioural therapy. *J Am Acad Child Adolesc Psychiatry*. **42**: 1279–85.

Biondi M and Picardi A (2005). Increased maintenance of obsessive compulsive disorder remission after integrated serotonergic and cognitive psychotherapy compared with medication alone. *Psychother Psychosom*. **74**: 123–8.

Boschen MJ, et al. (2008). Treatment of severe treatment-refractory obsessive–compulsive disorder: a study of inpatient and community treatment. *CNS Spectr*. **13**: 1056–65.

Buhlmann U, et al. (2006). Cognitive retraining for organisational impairment in obsessive–compulsive disorder. *Psychiatr Res*. **144**(2–3): 109–16

Calvocoressi L, et al. (1999). Family accommodation of obsessive–compulsive symptoms: instrument development and assessment of family behavior. *J Nerv Ment Dis*. **187**: 636–42.

Chamberlain SR and Sahakian BJ (2007). The neuropsychiatry of impulsivity. *Curr Opin Psychiatry*. **20**: 255–61.

Chamberlain SR, et al. (2005). The neuropsychology of obsessive compulsive disorder: the importance of failures in cognitive and behavioural inhibition as candidate endophenotypic markers. *Neurosci Biobehav Rev*. **29**: 399–419.

Chamberlain SR, et al. (2006). Motor inhibition and cognitive flexibility in obsessive–compulsive disorder and trichotillomania. *Am J Psychiatry*. **163**: 1282–4.

Chamberlain SR, et al. (2007a). Impaired cognitive flexibility and motor inhibition in first degree relatives of OCD patients: on the trail of endophenotypes. *Am J Psychiatry*. **164**: 335–8.

Chamberlain SR, et al. (2007b). A neuropsychological comparison of obsessive–compulsive disorder and trichotillomania. *Neuropsychologia*. **45**: 654–62.

Chamberlain SR, et al. (2008). Orbitofrontal dysfunction in patients with obsessive–compulsive disorder and their unaffected relatives. *Science*. **321**: 421–2.

Cottraux J, et al. (1990). A controlled study of fluvoxamine and exposure in obsessive–compulsive disorder. *Int Clin Psychopharmacol*. **5**: 17–30.

Cuijpers P, et al. (2014). Adding psychotherapy to antidepressant medication in depression and anxiety disorders: a meta-analysis. *World Psychiatry*. **13**: 56–67.

de Houwer J, et al. (2001). Association learning of likes and dislikes: a review of 25 years of research on human evaluative conditioning. *Psychol Bull*. **127**: 853–69.

de Vries FE, et al. (2014). Compensatory frontoparietal activity during working memory: an endophenotype of obsessive–compulsive disorder. *Biol Psychiatry*. **76**: 878–87.

Dingemans AE, et al. (2014).The effectiveness of cognitive remediation therapy in patients with a severe or enduring eating disorder: a randomised controlled trial. *Psychother Psychosom*. **83**: 29–36.

Fineberg NA and Gale TM (2005). Evidence-based pharmacotherapy of obsessive–compulsive disorder. *Int J Neuropsychopharmacol*. **8**: 107–29.

Fineberg NA, *et al.* (1997). Brain 5-HT function in obsessive–compulsive disorder. Prolactin responses to d-fenfluramine. *Br J Psychiatry*. **171**: 280–2.

Fineberg NA, *et al.* (2010). Probing compulsive and impulsive behaviors, from animal models to endophenotypes: a narrative review. *Neuropsychopharmacology*. **35**: 591–604.

Fineberg NA, *et al.* (2014). New developments in human neurocognition: clinical, genetic, and brain imaging correlates of impulsivity and compulsivity. *CNS Spectr*. **19**: 69–89.

Flessner CA, *et al.* (2010).The impact of neuropsychological functioning on treatment outcome in pediatric obsessive–compulsive disorder. *Depress Anxiety*. **27**: 365–71.

Foa EB, *et al.* (2013). Six-month follow-up of a randomized controlled trial augmenting serotonin reuptake inhibitor treatment with exposure and ritual prevention for obsessive–compulsive disorder. *J Clin Psychiatry*. **74**: 464–9.

Freeman J, *et al.* (2014). Family-based treatment of early childhood obsessive–compulsive disorder: the Pediatric Obsessive–Compulsive Disorder Treatment Study for Young Children (POTS Jr)—a randomized clinical trial. *JAMA Psychiatry*. **71**: 689–98.

Freud S (1926). *Inhibitions, symptoms, and anxiety*. Standard Edition. **20**: 111–31.

Gillan CM, *et al.* (2014). Enhanced avoidance habits in obsessive–compulsive disorder. *Biol Psychiatry*. **75**: 631–8.

Greist JH (1994). Behavior therapy for obsessive compulsive disorder. *J Clin Psychiatry*. **55** (Suppl): 60–8.

Griffiths F, *et al.* (2006). Why are health care interventions delivered over the internet? A systematic review of the published literature. *J Med Internet Res*. **8**: e10.

Helbig-Lang S and Peterman F (2010). Tolerate or eliminate? A systematic review on the effects of safety behaviors across anxiety disorders. *Clin Psychol: Sci Pr*. **17**: 218–33.

Hohagen F, *et al.* (1998). Combination of behaviour therapy with fluvoxamine in comparison with behaviour therapy and placebo: results of a multi-centre study. *Br J Psychiatry*. **173** (Suppl. 35): 71–8.

Hollander E and Cohen LJ (1996). The psychobiology and psychopharmacology of compulsive spectrum disorders. In: Oldham J, Hollander E, Skodol A, eds. *Impulsivity and Compulsivity*. Washington DC: American Psychiatric Press, Inc., pp. 143–66.

Hollander E, *et al.* (1992). Serotonergic function in obsessive–compulsive disorder: behavioural and neuroendocrine responses to oral m-CPP and fenfluramine in patients and healthy volunteers. *Arch Gen Psychiatry*. **49**: 21–8.

Hollander E, *et al.* (1997). Psychosocial function and economic costs of obsessive–compulsive disorder. *CNS Spectrums*. **2**: 16–25.

Keeley ML, *et al.* (2008). Clinical predictors of response to cognitive-behavioral therapy for obsessive–compulsive disorder. *Clin Psychol Rev*. **28**: 118–30.

Lovinger DM (2010). Neurotransmitter roles in synaptic modulation, plasticity and learning in the dorsal striatum. *Neuropharmacol*. **58**: 951–61.

Macerollo A and Martino D (2013). Pediatric autoimmune neuropsychiatric disorders associated with streptococcal infections (PANDAS): an evolving concept. *Tremor Other Hyperkinet Mov (N Y)*. **3**. pii: tre-03-167-4158-7. eCollection 2013.

March JS, *et al.* (1994). Behavioural psychotherapy for children and adolescents with obsessive–compulsive disorder: an open trial of a new protocol driven treatment package. *J Am Acad Child Adolesc Psychiatry*. **33**: 333–41.

March JS, *et al.* (2001). Cognitive-behavioural psychotherapy for pediatric obsessive–compulsive disorder. *J Clin Child Psychol*. **30**: 8–18.

March J.S, *et al.* (2006). Treatment benefits and the risk of suicidality in multi-centre randomised controlled trials of sertraline in children and adolescents. *Child Adolsc Psychopharmacol*. **16** (1–2): 91–102.

Marks I (1997). Behaviour therapy for obsessive–compulsive disorder: a decade of progress. *Can J Psychiatry*. **42**: 1021–7.

Marks IM, *et al.* (1980). Clomipramine and exposure for obsessive–compulsive rituals. *Br J Psychiatry*. **136**: 1–25.

Marks IM, *et al.* (1988). Clomipramine, self exposure and therapist aided exposure for obsessive–compulsive rituals. *Br J Psychiatry*. **152**: 522–34.

Martin LJ, *et al.* (1991). Social deprivation of infant monkeys alters the chemoarchitecture of the brain: I. Subcortical regions. *J Neurosci*. **11**: 3344–58.

Mawson D, *et al.* (1982). Clomipramine and exposure for chronic obsessive–compulsive rituals: two-year follow-up and further findings. *Br J Psychiatry*. **140**: 11–18.

McDougle CJ, *et al.* (2000). A double-blind, placebo-controlled study of risperidone addition in serotonin reuptake inhibitor–refractory obsessive–compulsive disorder. *Arch Gen Psychiatry*. **57**: 794–801.

Menzies L, *et al.* (2007). Neurocognitive endophenotypes of obsessive–compulsive disorder. *Brain*. **130** (Pt 12): 3223–36.

Milad MR and Rauch SL (2012). Obsessive–compulsive disorder: beyond segregated cortico-striatal pathways. *Trends Cogn Sci*. **16**: 43–51.

Moritz S, *et al.* (2005). Neurocognitive impairment does not predict treatment outcome in obsessive–compulsive disorder. *Behav Res Ther*. 43: 811–19.

Naqvi NH, Rudrauf D, Damasio H, and Bechara A (2007). Damage to the insula disrupts addiction to cigarette smoking. *Science*. **315**: 531.

National Institute for Health and Care Excellence (2005). Clinical guideline 31. Obsessive–compulsive disorder: core interventions in the treatment of obsessive–compulsive disorder and body dysmorphic disorder. Available at: <http://www.NICE.org.uk/cg31>.

Neziroglu F, *et al.* (2004). Overvalued ideation as a predictor of fluvoxamine response in patients with OCD. *Psychiatry Res*. **125**: 53–60.

Nicholson TR, *et al.* (2012). Prevalence of anti-basal ganglia antibodies in adult obsessive–compulsive disorder: cross-sectional study. *Br J Psychiatry*. **200**: 381–6.

Obsessive Compulsive Cognitions Working Group (1997). Cognitive assessment of obsessive–compulsive disorder. *Behav Res Ther*. **35**: 667–81.

Park HS, *et al.* (2006). Effects of cognitive training focusing on organisational strategies in patients with obsessive–compulsive disorder. *Psychiatry Clin Neurosci*. **60**: 355–60.

Pinto A, *et al.* (2011). Obsessive compulsive personality disorder as a predictor of exposure and ritual prevention outcome for obsessive compulsive disorder. *Behav Res Ther*. **49**: 453–8.

Pinto A, *et al.* (2013). Development and preliminary psychometric evaluation of a self-rated version of the Family Accommodation Scale for Obsessive–Compulsive Disorder. *J Obsessive Compuls Relat Disord*. **2**: 457–65.

Porto PR, *et al.* (2009). Does cognitive behavioural therapy change the brain? A systematic review of neuroimaging in anxiety disorders. *J Neuropsychiatry Clin Neurosci*. **21**: 114–25.

Potenza MN (2007). To do or not to do? The complexities of addiction, motivation, self-control, and impulsivity. *Am J Psychiatry*. **164**: 4–6.

Purdon C (2008). Unacceptable obsessional thoughts and covert rituals. In: Abramowitz JS, McKay D, and Taylor S, eds. *Clinical handbook of obsessive–compulsive disorder and related problems*. Baltimore: Johns Hopkins University Press, pp. 61–75.

Radomsky A, *et al.* (2010). Cognitive-behavior therapy for compulsive checking in OCD. *Cogn Behav Pract*. **17**: 119–31.

Rapoport JL (1989). *The boy who couldn't stop washing: the experience and treatment of obsessive–compulsive disorder*. New York: EP Dutton.

Rauch SL, *et al.* (1997). Probing striatal function in obsessive–compulsive disorder: a PET study of implicit sequence learning. *J Neuropsychiatry Clin Neurosci*. **9**: 568–73.

Robbins TW and Brown VJ (1990). The role of the striatum in the mental chronometry of action: a theoretical review. *Rev Neurosci*. **2**: 181–213.

Salkovskis PM (1999). Understanding and treating obsessive–compulsive disorder. *Behav Res Ther*. **37** (suppl). 29–52.

Saxena S and Rauch SL (2000). Functional neuroimaging and the neuroanatomy of obsessive–compulsive disorder. *Psychiatr Clin North Am*. **23**: 563–86.

Simpson HB, *et al.* (2004). Post-treatment effects of exposure therapy and clomipramine in obsessive–compulsive disorder. *Depress Anxiety*. **19**: 225–33.

Simpson HB, *et al.* (2008). A randomized controlled trial of cognitive-behavioral therapy for augmenting pharmacotherapy in obsessive–compulsive disorder. *Am J Psychiatry*. **165**: 621–30.

Simpson HB, *et al.* (2013). Cognitive-behavioral therapy vs risperidone for augmenting serotonin reuptake inhibitors in obsessive–compulsive disorder: a randomized clinical trial. *JAMA Psychiatry*. **70**: 1190–9.

Sookman D and Steketee G (2007). Directions in specialized cognitive behavior therapy for resistant obsessive compulsive disorder: Theory and practice of two approaches. *Cogn Behav Pract*. **14**: 1–17. In special issue: Advances and future directions in cognitive behavior therapy for resistant anxiety disorders, Sookman D, guest editor.

Sookman D, et al. (2003). Role of dysfunctional beliefs on efficacy of CBT for resistant OCD. Paper presented at the 37th annual convention of Association for Advancement of Behavior Therapy. Boston, MA.

Stein DJ (1997). Psychiatry on the Internet: Survey of an OCD mailing list. *Psychiatric Bull*. **21**: 95–9.

Stein DJ and Hollander E (1993). Neurobiology of impulsivity and the impulse control disorders. *Neurosciences*. **5**: 9–17.

Stein DJ and Hollander E (1993). Impulsive aggression and obsessive–compulsive disorder. *Psychiatric Annals*. **23**: 389–95.

Stein DJ and Rapoport JL (1996). Cross-cultural studies and obsessive–compulsive disorder. *CNS Spectr*. **1**: 42–6.

Stein DJ and Stone MH (1997). *Essential papers on obsessive–compulsive disorders*. New York: New York University Press.

Stein DJ, et al. (1999). Single photon emission computed tomography of the brain with Tc-99m HMPAO during sumatriptan challenge in obsessive–compulsive disorder: investigating the functional role of the serotonin auto-receptor. *Prog Neuropsychopharmacol Biol Psychiatry*. **23**: 1079–99.

Stein DJ, et al. (2001). An integrated approach to the treatment of OCD. In: Fineberg N, Marazziti D, and Stein DJ, eds. *Obsessive–compulsive disorder: a practical guide*. London: Martin Seedat.

Summerfeldt LJ (2004). Understanding and treating incompleteness in obsessive–compulsive disorder. *J Clin Psychol*. **60**: 1155–68.

Swedo SE and Grant PJ (2005). Annotation: PANDAS: a model for human autoimmune disease. *J Child Psychol Psychiat Allied Discipl*. **46**: 227–34.

Swedo SE, et al. (1992). Cerebral glucose metabolism in childhood-onset obsessive–compulsive disorder: revisualization during pharmacotherapy. *Arch Gen Psychiatry*. **49**: 690–4.

Swedo SE, et al. (1998). Pediatric autoimmune neuropsychiatric disorders associated with streptococcal infections: clinical description of the first 50 cases. *Am J Psychiat*. **155**: 264–71.

Tallis F (1995). *Obsessive–compulsive disorder, a cognitive and neuro-psychological perspective*. Chilester: John Wiley and Sons Ltd.

Thornicroft G, et al. (1991). An in-patient behavioural psychotherapy unit. Description and audit. *Br J Psychiatry*. **158**: 362–7.

Tolin DF, et al. (2006). Are obsessive beliefs specific to OCD?: a comparison across anxiety disorders. *Behav Res Ther*. **44**: 469–80.

van Balkom AJLM, et al. (1994). A meta-analysis on the treatment of obsessive–compulsive disorder: a comparison of antidepressants, behavior, and cognitive therapy. *Clin Psychol Rev*. **14**: 359–81.

van den Heuvel OA, et al. (2005). Frontal-striatal dysfunction during planning in obsessive–compulsive disorder. *Arch Gen Psychiatry*. **62**: 301–9.

Vriend C, et al. (2013). Switch the itch: a naturalistic follow-up study on the neural correlates of cognitive flexibility in obsessive–compulsive disorder. *Psychiatry Res*. **213**: 31–8.

Wells A (2011). *Metacognitive therapy for anxiety and depression*. New York: Guilford.

Whiteside SP, et al. (2004). A meta-analysis of functional neuroimaging in obsessive–compulsive disorder. *Psychiatry Res*. **132**: 69–79.

Whittal ML., et al. (2005). Treatment of obsessive–compulsive disorder: cognitive behavior therapy versus exposure with response prevention. *Behav Res Ther*. **43**: 1559–76.

Zitterl W, et al. (2000). Naturalistic course of obsessive–compulsive disorder and comorbid depression: longitudinal results of a prospective follow-up study of 74 actively treated patients. *Psychopathology*. **33**: 75–80.

Zohar J, et al. (1987). Serotonergic responsivity in obsessive–compulsive disorder: comparison of patients and healthy controls. *Arch Gen Psychiatry*. **44**: 946–51.

Zor R, et al. (2011). Manifestation of incompleteness in obsessive–compulsive disorder (OCD) as reduced functionality and extended activity beyond task completion. *PLoS One*. **6**: e25217.

# Further reading

Cuijpers P, *et al*. (2014). Adding psychotherapy to antidepressant medication in depression and anxiety disorders: a meta-analysis. *World Psychiatry*. **13**: 56–67.

Hohagen F, *et al*. (1998). Combination of behaviour therapy with fluvoxamine in comparison with behaviour therapy and placebo: results of a multi-centre study. *Br J Psychiatry*. **173** (Suppl. 35): 71–8

Rauch SL and Baxter LR Jr (1998). Neuroimaging in obsessive–compulsive disorder and related disorders: In: Jenicke MA, Baer L, Minichiello WE, eds. *Obsessive–compulsive disorders: practical management*, 3rd edition. St Louis: Mosby, pp. 289–317.

Simpson HB, *et al*. (2008). A randomized controlled trial of cognitive-behavioral therapy for augmenting pharmacotherapy in obsessive–compulsive disorder. *Am J Psychiatry*. **165**: 621–30.

Stein DJ and Stone MH (1997). *Essential papers on obsessive–compulsive disorders*. New York: New York University Press.

# Chapter 6

# Conclusion

This volume has covered the phenomenology, psychobiology, pharmacotherapy, and psychotherapy of OCD. We have also briefly considered some of the OCD-related conditions. We have attempted to synthesize the growing research literature, with the aim of providing practical guidance to clinicians.

Significant advances have been made in describing the complex phenomenology of OCD, and this has important practical implications. First, given the high prevalence of OCD and related conditions, there is growing consensus that there is value in screening patients with simple questions such as those listed by Zohar and Fineberg (see Box 2.1, Chapter 2). A high index of suspicion for OCD is justified in a number of contexts, including dermatology clinics, patients with tics, and pregnancy. Additional work is needed to reverse the underdiagnosis and undertreament of OCD.

Second, there is again a good deal of consensus that only a few symptom dimensions capture much of the variance in OCD symptoms. Of course, it is important for clinicians to remain on the lookout for rarer forms of OCD. Instruments, such as the DY-BOCS, which focus on four key symptom dimensions, appear to be useful in the clinical setting. Instruments are also available for the assessment of OCD symptoms in children and adolescents.

Third, many authors have emphasized that OCD overlaps phenomenologically and psychobiologically with conditions such as Tourette's syndrome and BDD, whereas it has less in common with the anxiety disorders. Although the concept of the 'OCD spectrum' requires further research and validation, it has immediate utility in the clinical setting. In particular, patients with OCD should be screened for OCD and related disorders, which are now classified in their own chapter in DSM-5.

In Chapter 3, on the pathogenesis of OCD, we emphasized the value of a CSTC model for conceptualizing the psychobiology of OCD. A focus on the CSTC circuitry allows an integration of several different sets of data on OCD, ranging from cognitive and affective studies, through to brain imaging research, and on to more molecular work on this disorder. In addition, a focus on the CSTC circuitry provides a basis for integrating work on the pharmacotherapy, psychotherapy, and neurosurgical treatment of OCD.

We can briefly review some of these data here. First, involvement of the CSTC circuitry in OCD is useful in understanding studies on the neuropsychiatry and neuropsychology of OCD. These have demonstrated an association between OCD and motoric symptoms (such as tics), cognitive disruptions (e.g. impairment in implicit learning, cognitive inflexibility), and affective dysregulation (e.g. impairments in the processing of emotion, impaired inhibition). Some of these disruptions may have a strong genetic component and may comprise endophenotypic vulnerabilities to OCD. The striatum mediates a broad range of motoric, cognitive, and affective functions, consistent with the range of impairments found in OCD and related conditions.

Second, involvement of the CSTC circuitry is useful in integrating data on structural, functional, and molecular imaging in OCD. Although structural findings have documented involvement of the striatum in OCD, it is possible that increased volume is seen during acute episodes of PANDAS, while decreased volumes are characteristic of more chronic disease. Functional imaging studies have demonstrated increased activity at rest, and especially during symptom provocation, in the CSTC circuitry. Cognitive and affective paradigms (e.g. implicit learning) also demonstrate disruption of CSTC function in OCD. There is increased interest in brain imaging endophenotypic markers for OCD.

Third, there is a growing understanding of the specific molecular alterations found in the CSTC circuitry, which may be associated with OCD. Genetic studies have indicated that some patients with OCD have rare functional variations in the SERT in serotonergic neurons that play a key role in the striatum. Studies of dopamine receptor binding have also demonstrated abnormalities in the basal ganglia circuitry in OCD. Magnetic resonance spectroscopy has indicated alterations in the glutamatergic system in the CSTC circuitry in OCD.

Fourth, a CSTC model is useful in providing an integrated understanding of different therapeutic approaches to OCD. Pharmacotherapy, psychotherapy, and neurosurgery all result in a normalization of the dysfunction in the CSTC circuitry that is so characteristic of OCD. Nevertheless, it appears that pharmacotherapy and psychotherapy have different predictors of response; thus, each may exert its effect in a unique way. Although the combination of pharmacotherapy and psychotherapy does not always yield a more robust response than either modality alone, there is a theoretical rationale for using both forms of treatment together, and there is a growing empirical database of studies which support this strategy.

Finally, we have reviewed current knowledge of the pharmacotherapy and psychotherapy of OCD. Meta-analyses of the RCTs in OCD have clearly demonstrated that SSRIs are the medication treatment of choice, while CBT (with ERP) is the psychotherapy of choice in OCD. The efficacy of SSRIs and CBT is clear not only in adults, but also in children and adolescents with OCD.

Several consensus documents have been published on OCD. The Cape Town consensus emphasized that SSRIs are the first choice of medication in OCD, and subsequent guidelines have again emphasized this point (Koran and Simpson 2013). It noted that these agents may need to be given at a higher dose and for a longer duration than is usually the case in disorders such as depression. The SSRIs are useful not only for OCD, but also for a range of obsessive-compulsive spectrum disorders (Box 6.1). Finally, patients with OCD not only respond to medication, but some also experience significant improvement in symptoms, and sometimes even remission.

In the management of refractory patients, a number of key principles must be underlined. Diagnosis should be reconsidered, and general medical conditions excluded. Medication history should be carefully reviewed, and adherence to medication established. Dopamine blockers are currently the pharmacotherapy augmentation strategy of choice (Ducasse *et al.*

---

### Box 6.1 OCD spectrum disorders that may respond to SSRIs

- BDD
- Hoarding disorder
- Hypochondriasis
- Obsessive-compulsive symptoms in autistic disorder
- Obsessive-compulsive symptoms in intellectual disability
- Obsessive-compulsive symptoms in Tourette's disorder
- Olfactory reference syndrome
- Onychophagia (severe nail biting)
- Skin-picking (excoriation) disorder
- Trichotillomania (hair-pulling disorder)

2014) and should be effective in around 50% of patients. In those patients who fail to respond to a range of SSRIs and augmentation strategies, more unusual interventions can be considered (including intravenous clomipramine, supraformulary doses of SRIs, rTMS, DBS, and stereo-tactic neurosurgery).

A final crucial component of treatment is psycho-education. Consumer advocacy groups have played a vital role in increasing awareness of this disorder in the community and in encouraging early diagnosis and treatment. The Internet provides a number of excellent resources for OCD patients, and a number of virtual support groups are useful for some patients. Additional work is needed to improve mental health literacy in general, and knowledge of OCD in particular.

Taken together, advances in understanding the phenomenology, psychobiology, pharmaco-therapy, and psychotherapy of OCD have improved the prognosis of those diagnosed with OCD. Nevertheless, much remains to be learned about this intriguing and complex disor-der. We are hopeful that, as further strides are made in understanding the psychobiology of OCD, so additional interventions will be developed and the prognosis of this disorder further improved. Advances in a range of clinical neuroscience methodologies raise the possibility that ultimately clinicians will be able to approach the assessment and treatment of OCD using a personalized medicine approach. In the interim, much can be done for patients with OCD, using available technologies.

# References

Ducasse D, *et al*. (2014). D2 and D3 dopamine receptor affinity predicts effectiveness of antipsychotic drugs in obsessive–compulsive disorders: a metaregression analysis. *Psychopharmacology (Berl)*. **231**: 3765–70.

Koran LM and Simpson HB (2013). *Guideline Watch (March 2013): Practice Guideline for the Treatment of Patients With Obsessive–Compulsive Disorder*. Washington, DC: American Psychiatric Association. <http://psychiatryonline.org/pb/assets/raw/sitewide/practice_guidelines/guidelines/ocd-watch.pdf> (accessed 7 March 2015).

# Resources for patients and clinicians and major rating scales for OCD

# Appendix 1

# Resources for patients and clinicians

## Major rating scales for obsessive-compulsive disorder

| Y-BOCS | (see p. 91) |
|--------|-------------|
| CY-BOCS | (see p. 105) |
| DY-BOCS | (see p. 119) |
| CGI | (see p. 139) |
| Z-FOCS | (see p. 8) |

## Information and self-help books for children and adults with obsessive-compulsive disorder, body dysmorphic disorder, and trichotillomania, and their carers

Patients and their carers can benefit greatly from guided self-help, using educational books and treatment manuals. There are a number of publications available. Below are just a few that the authors have found to be helpful.

### Obsessive-compulsive disorder

*Children*

Wagner P and Pinto A (2000). *Up and down the worry hill: a children's book about obsessive compulsive disorder and its treatment.* Lighthouse Point, FL: Lighthouse Press.

An illustrated book designed to help parents and professionals explain OCD to children through the story of 'Casey', a young boy with OCD.

Wever C and Phillips N (1996). *The secret problem.*

A cartoon book that describes OCD in clear and simple language to help children, teenagers, and parents understand OCD and its treatment.

*Adults and older adolescents*

Adam D (2014). *The man who couldn't stop: OCD and the true story of a life lost in thought.* London: Picador.

Royal College of Psychiatrists (2014). *Obsessive-compulsive disorder: mental health information for all.* Available at: <http://www.rcpsych.ac.uk/healthadvice/problemsdisorders/obsessivecompulsivedisorder.aspx>.

Challacombe F, et al. (2011). *Break free from OCD: overcoming obsessive compulsive disorder with CBT.* London: Vermilion.

Hyman B and Pedrick C (2005). *The OCD workbook: your guide to breaking free from obsessive-compulsive disorder.* Oakland, CA: New Harbinger Publications.

A self-treatment manual for adults and older adolescents that guides the person with OCD through ERP, with advice for family members.

Schwartz JM (1997). *Brain lock: free yourself from obsessive compulsive behavior*. New York: HarperCollins.
A self-treatment manual suitable for adults and older adolescents with OCD.

Veale D and Willson R (2005). *Overcoming obsessive compulsive disorder*. London: Constable & Robinson.
A self-treatment book suitable for adults and older teenagers.

Tallis F (1992). *Understanding obsessions and compulsions: a self-help manual*. London: Sheldon Press.
A self-treatment book suitable for adults and older teenagers.

Rapaport J (1989). *The boy who couldn't stop washing: the experience and treatment of OCD*. New York: Plume Books.
Seminal text describing the experience and treatment of OCD.

## Body dysmorphic disorder

Wilson R, *et al.* (2009). *Overcoming body image problems, including body dysmorphic disorder*. London: Robinson.

Philips K (1996). *The broken mirror: understanding and treating body dysmorphic disorder*. Oxford: Oxford University Press.
Describes the experience of BDD and discusses self-assessment, CBT, and medication.

Claiborn J and Pedrick C (2002). *The BDD workbook: overcome body dysmorphic disorder and end body image obsessions*. Oakland, CA: New Harbinger Publications.
A self-treatment book suitable for adults and older teenagers.

## Trichotillomania

Penzel F (2003). *The hair-pulling problem: a complete guide to trichotillomania*. Oxford: Oxford University Press.
Includes information on setting up a self-treatment programme with a section for parents.

Keuthen N, *et al.* (2001). *Help for hairpullers: understanding and coping with trichotillomania*. Oakland, CA: New Harbinger Publications.
A self-treatment book suitable for adults and older teenagers.

## Tourette's syndrome

Buffolano S (2012). *Coping with Tourette syndrome: a workbook for kids with tic disorders*. Oakland, CA: New Harbinger Publications.

Bruun RD and Bruun B (1994). *A mind of its own: Tourette's syndrome: a story and a guide*. Oxford: Oxford University Press.
Describes the experience of Tourette's. Suitable for adults and older teenagers.

## Hypochondriasis

Scheitzer P, *et al.* (2010). *Help for hypochondriasis: a guide to understanding treatment and resources*. Raleigh, NC: Lulu.com.

Cantor C and Fallon B (1997). *Phantom illness: recognizing, understanding, and overcoming hypochondria*. New York: Houghton Mifflin
Autobiography, covering one woman's struggle with hypochondriasis and including many case examples and treatment strategies.

## Hoarding disorder

Tolin DF, *et al.* (2007). *Buried in treasures: help for compulsive acquiring, saving and hoarding*. Cary, NC: Oxford University Press.

## Skin-picking disorder

Pasternak A and Fletcher T (2014). *Skin picking: the freedom to finally stop*. Annette Pasternak.

Florendale D (2011). *The complete guide to compulsive skin picking disorders*. CreateSpace Independent Publishing Platform. Available at: <https://www.createspace.com>.

# Information for health care practitioners

Clinicians may also benefit from reading the following.

## Obsessive-compulsive disorder

Grant J, et al. (2015). *Clinical guide to obsessive compulsive and related disorders.* Oxford: Oxford University Press.

A comprehensive overview of OCD and related disorders (trichotillomania, excoriation disorder, hoarding disorder, BDD, and tic disorders). The book covers the underlying causes, clinical presentations, and treatments.

Storch E and Mckay D, eds. (2014). *Obsessive-compulsive disorder and its spectrum: a lifespan approach.* Washington DC: American Psychological Association.

This book reviews the latest research on OCD and spectrum disorders and provides evidence-based guidance for assessment and treatment.

Zohar J, ed. (2012). *Obsessive compulsive disorder: current science and clinical practice (World Psychiatric Association).* Hoboken, NJ: Wiley-Blackwell.

This book focuses on recent information on biological mechanisms, assessment, diagnosis, and treatment of OCD.

Fineberg N, et al., eds (2001). *Obsessive compulsive disorder: a practical guide.* London: Martin Dunitz.

A practical guide for clinicians covering the aetiology and treatment (CBT, medication, and other forms of treatment).

Fineberg N and Nigam A. *Obsessive-compulsive disorder: a guide to recognition and management. BMJ Online Learning.* Available at: <<http://learning.bmj.com/learning/module-intro/obsessive-compulsive-disorder-recognition-management.html?moduleId=5004330&searchTerm= "Fineberg N and Nigam A. Obsessive-compulsive disorder: a guide to recognition and management. "&page=1&locale=en_GB> (accessed 7 March 2015).

Online resource for medical practitioners and allied professionals interested in learning more about the recognition and clinical treatments for OCD.

Foa EF, et al. (1998). *OCD in children and adolescents: a cognitive-behavioural treatment manual.* New York: Guilford Press.

A manualized approach to CBT treatment of OCD, including psycho-educational material and questionnaires.

Clark DA (2003). *Cognitive behavioural therapy for OCD.* New York: Guilford Press.

Overview of cognitive and behavioural techniques for the treatment of OCD.

Heyman I, et al. (2006). Obsessive-compulsive disorder. *BMJ.* **333**: 424–9.

Contemporary review for medical practitioners and allied professionals interested in the neurobiological theories and clinical treatments for OCD.

## Body dysmorphic disorder

Grant J, et al. (2014). *Clinical guide to obsessive compulsive and related disorders.* Oxford: Oxford University Press.

A comprehensive overview of OCD and related disorders (trichotillomania, excoriation disorder, hoarding disorder, BDD, and tic disorders). The book covers the underlying causes, clinical presentations, and treatments.

Storch E and Mckay D, eds. (2014). *Obsessive-compulsive disorder and its spectrum: a lifespan approach.* Washington DC: American Psychological Association.

This book reviews the latest research on OCD and spectrum disorders and provides evidence-based guidance for the assessment and treatment of spectrum disorders.

Steketee G, ed. (2011). *The Oxford handbook of obsessive compulsive and spectrum disorders.* Carey, NC: Oxford University Press.

This handbook reviews the recent literature on OCD and associated spectrum conditions.

Philips K (1996). *The broken mirror: understanding and treating body dysmorphic disorder.* Oxford: Oxford University Press.

Describes the experience of BDD and discusses self-assessment, CBT approaches, and medication.

## Trichotillomania

Grant J, et al. (2014). *Clinical guide to obsessive compulsive and related disorders.* Oxford: Oxford University Press.

A comprehensive overview of OCD and related disorders (trichotillomania, excoriation disorder, hoarding disorder, BDD, and tic disorders). The book covers the underlying causes, clinical presentations, and treatments.

Storch E and Mckay D, eds. (2014). *Obsessive-compulsive disorder and its spectrum: a lifespan approach.* Washington DC: American Psychological Association

This book reviews the latest research on OCD and spectrum disorders and provides evidence-based guidance for the assessment and treatment of spectrum disorders.

Steketee G, ed. (2011). *The Oxford handbook of obsessive compulsive and spectrum disorders.* Carey, NC: Oxford University Press.

This handbook reviews recent literature on OCD and associated spectrum conditions.

Franklin ME and Tolin DF (2007). *Treating trichotillomania: cognitive–behavioural therapy for hairpulling and related problems.* New York: Springer.

A comprehensive clinical- and empirical-based volume which covers biopsychosocial theories, assessment, diagnosis, and treatment of trichotillomania.

Stein D, et al. (1999). *Trichotillomania.* Arlington: American Psychiatric Publishing.

Describes the evaluation and treatment of compulsive hair-pulling.

## Hoarding disorder

Grant J, et al. (2014). *Clinical guide to obsessive compulsive and related disorders.* Oxford: Oxford University Press

A comprehensive overview of OCD and related disorders (trichotillomania, excoriation disorder, hoarding disorder, BDD, and tic disorders). The book covers the underlying causes, clinical presentations, and treatments.

Storch E and Mckay D. eds. (2014). *Obsessive-compulsive disorder and its spectrum: a lifespan approach.* Washington DC: American Psychological Association

This book reviews the latest research on OCD and spectrum disorders and provides evidence-based guidance for the assessment and treatment of spectrum disorders.

Steketee G and Frost RO (2013). *Treatment for hoarding disorder: workbook: treatments that work.* Carey, NC: Oxford University Press.

Steketee G ed. (2011). *The Oxford handbook of obsessive compulsive and spectrum disorders.* Carey, NC: Oxford University Press.

This handbook reviews recent literature on OCD and associated spectrum conditions.

## Tourette's syndrome and tic disorders

Grant J, et al. (2014). *Clinical guide to obsessive compulsive and related disorders.* Oxford: Oxford University Press.

A comprehensive overview of OCD and related disorders (trichotillomania, excoriation disorder, hoarding disorder, BDD, and tic disorders). The book covers the underlying causes, clinical presentations, and treatments.

Storch E and Mckay D, eds. (2014). *Obsessive-compulsive disorder and its spectrum: a lifespan approach.* Washington DC: American Psychological Association.

This book reviews the latest research on OCD and spectrum disorders and provides evidence-based guidance for the assessment and treatment for spectrum disorders.

Steketee G ed. (2011). *The Oxford handbook of obsessive compulsive and spectrum disorders*. Carey, NC: Oxford University Press.

This handbook reviews recent literature on OCD and associated spectrum conditions.

### Skin-picking disorder

Grant J, et al. (2014). *Clinical guide to obsessive compulsive and related disorders*. Oxford: Oxford University Press.

A comprehensive overview of OCD and related disorders (trichotillomania, excoriation disorder, hoarding disorder, BDD, and tic disorders). The book covers the underlying causes, clinical presentations, and treatments.

Storch E and Mckay D, eds. (2014). *Obsessive-compulsive disorder and its spectrum: a lifespan approach*. Washington DC: American Psychological Association.

This book reviews the latest research on OCD and spectrum disorders and provides evidence-based guidance for the assessment and treatment for spectrum disorders.

## Useful websites for clinicians and patients

<http://www.icocs.org>
International College of Obsessive Compulsive Spectrum Disorders (ICOCS). Charity aimed at promoting collaborative research and raising the profile of OCD and obsessive-compulsive related disorders. Membership includes researchers, practitioners, individuals with OCD, and their carers.

<http://www.ocdyouth.info>
Information on OCD and how to recover for young people and their carers.

<http://iocdf.org/>
International OCD Foundation.

<http://www.nice.org.uk>
Website for NICE guidelines.

<http://www.BAP.org.uk>
Website for BAP guidelines on anxiety disorders (including OCD).

## Consumer associations involved in obsessive-compulsive disorder

### Australia

Anxiety Disorders Foundation of Australia, Inc.
<http://www.connectingup.org/organisation/anxiety-disorders-foundation-of-australia-inc-nsw>

Anxiety Recovery Centre Victoria
<https://www.arcvic.org.au/>

Anxiety & Stress Management Service of Australia
<http://www.anxietyhelp.com.au/>

### Canada

The Ontario Obsessive Compulsive Disorder Network (OOCDN)
<http://www.ocdontario.org/>

### South Africa

Obsessive-Compulsive Disorder Association of South Africa

PO Box 87127, Houghton, 2041, South Africa. Tel: (+2711) 786–7030. Fax: (+2711) 786 5866

## United Kingdom

OCD Action
<http://www.ocdaction.org.uk>

OCD-UK
<http://www.ocduk.org/>

First Steps to Freedom
<http://www.first-steps.org/>

## United States

International OCD Foundation.
<http://iocdf.org/>

National Tourette Syndrome Association
<http://www.tsa-usa.org/>

# Guidelines for treatment in obsessive-compulsive disorder

## American Psychiatric Association (APA) guidelines

Koran LM, et al. (2007). *Practice guideline for the treatment of patients with obsessive-compulsive disorder.* Arlington: American Psychiatric Association. Available at: <http://psychiatryonline.org/pb/assets/raw/sitewide/practice_guidelines/guidelines/ocd.pdf>.

Koran LM and Simpson HB (2013). *Guideline Watch: Practice Guideline for the Treatment of Patients With Obsessive-Compulsive Disorder.* Available at: <http://psychiatryonline.org/pb/assets/raw/sitewide/practice_guidelines/guidelines/ocd-watch.pdf>.

## British Association of Psychopharmacology guidelines

Baldwin DS, et al. (2014). Evidence-based pharmacological treatment of anxiety disorders, post-traumatic stress disorder and obsessive-compulsive disorder: a revision of the 2005 guidelines from the British Association for Psychopharmacology. *J Psychopharmacol.* **28**:403–39.

## Canadian guidelines

The Canadian Anxiety Guidelines Initiative Group on behalf of the Anxiety Disorders Association of Canada (2014).

Katzman MA, et al. (2014). Canadian clinical practice guidelines for the management of anxiety, posttraumatic stress and obsessive-compulsive disorders. *BMC Psychiatry.* **14** (Suppl1): S1.

Canadian Psychiatric Association (2006). Clinical practice guidelines. Management of Anxiety Disorders. *Canadian J Psychiatry.* **51** (8 Suppl 2): 9S–91S.

## National Institute for Health and Care Excellence guidelines (NICE)

Obsessive-compulsive disorder Evidence Update September 2013. A summary of selected new evidence relevant to NICE clinical guideline 31 'Obsessive-compulsive disorder: core interventions in the treatment of obsessive-compulsive disorder and body dysmorphic disorder' (2005). Evidence Update 47. National Institute for Health and Care Excellence, Level 1A City Tower Piccadilly Plaza Manchester M1 4BT www.nice.org.uk. HYPERLINK "http://www.evidence.nhs.uk/evidence-update-47" www.evidence.nhs.uk/evidence-update-47. Sep 2013.

## The Cape Town consensus

Zohar J, et al. (2007). Consensus Statement. *CNS Spectr.* **2** (suppl. 3): 59–63.

## The Expert Consensus Panel for OCD

March JS, et al. (1997). The Expert Consensus Guideline series. Treatment of obsessive-compulsive disorder. *J Clin Psychiatry*. **58** (Suppl.): 1–72.

## The World Council on Anxiety

Greist JH, et al. (2003). Long-term treatment of obsessive-compulsive disorder in adults. *CNS Spectr*. **8**: 7–16.

## World Federation of Societies of Biological Psychiatry (WFSBP) guidelines

Bandelow B, Sher L, Bunevicius R, Hollander E, Kasper S, Zohar J, Möller HJ. (2012). Guidelines for the pharmacological treatment of anxiety disorders, obsessive-compulsive disorder and posttraumatic stress disorder in primary care. WFSBP Task Force on Mental Disorders in Primary Care; WFSBP Task Force on Anxiety Disorders, OCD and PTSD. Int J Psychiatry Clin Pract. 16(2):77–84.

Rothbart R, Amos T, Siegfried N, Ipser JC, Fineberg N, Chamberlain SR, Stein DJ.(2013). Cochrane Collaboration Review, Treatment of Trichotillomania. "http://www.ncbi.nlm.nih.gov/pubmed/24214100" Pharmacotherapy for trichotillomania. Cochrane Database Syst Rev. 8;11:CD007662. doi: 10.1002/14651858. CD007662.pub2.

# Appendix 2

# Yale–Brown Obsessive Compulsive Scale (Y-BOCS)

The Yale–Brown Obsessive Compulsive Scale (Y-BOCS) is a clinician-administered scale that assesses the type and severity of symptoms in patients with OCD. It is generally considered the best instrument currently available to clinicians for assessing treatment outcomes and symptom severity.

Y-BOCS is administered as a semi-structured interview and consists of a preliminary 64-item symptom checklist, followed by the main 19-item rating scale. The rating scale includes two main sub-scales—one measuring obsessions (items 1–5) and the other measuring compulsions (items 6–10)—which are used in determining the patient's total score. While the remaining items (11–19) are rated and may provide useful information to the clinician, they are not counted in the total score.

## Reference

Goodman WK, et al. (1989). The Yale-Brown Obsessive Compulsive Scale. I. Development, use and reliability. Arch Gen Psychiatry. **46**: 1006–11.

Clinicians interested in using this scale and/or obtaining the full instructions should contact Dr Wayne K. Goodman, Department of Psychiatry, University of Florida College of Medicine, PO Box 100256, Gainesville, FL 32610, USA.

Name _____     Date _____

Check all that apply, but clearly mark the principal symptoms with a 'P'.

(Rater must ascertain whether reported behaviours are bona fide symptoms of OCD, and not symptoms of another disorder such as simple phobia or hypochondriasis. Items marked * may or may not be OCD phenomena.)

Current   Past

### AGGRESSIVE OBSESSIONS

_____ _____  Fear might harm self

_____ _____  Fear might harm others

_____ _____  Violent or horrific images

_____ _____  Fear of blurting out obscenities or insults

_____ _____  Fear of doing something else embarrassing*

_____ _____  Fear will act on unwanted impulses (e.g. to stab friend)

_____ _____  Fear will steal things

_____ _____  Fear will harm others because not careful enough (e.g. hit/run motor vehicle accident)

_____ _____  Fear will be responsible for something else terrible happening (e.g. fire, burglary)

_____ _____  Other_____

### CONTAMINATION OBSESSIONS

_____ _____  Concerns or disgust with bodily waste or secretions (e.g. urine, faeces, saliva)

_____ _____  Concern with dirt or germs

_____ _____  Excessive concern with environmental contaminants (e.g. asbestos, radiation, toxic waste)

_____ _____  Excessive concern with household items (e.g. cleansers, solvents)

_____ _____  Excessive concern with animals (e.g. insects)

_____ _____  Bothered by sticky substances or residues

_____ _____  Concerned will get ill because of contaminant

_____ _____  Concerned will get others ill by spreading contaminant (aggressive)

_____ _____  No concern with consequences of contamination other than how it might feel

_____ _____  Other_____

## SEXUAL OBSESSIONS

| | | |
|---|---|---|
| _____ | _____ | Forbidden or perverse sexual thoughts, images, or impulses |
| _____ | _____ | Content involves children or incest |
| _____ | _____ | Content involves homosexuality* |
| _____ | _____ | Sexual behaviour toward others (aggressive)* |
| _____ | _____ | Other_____ |

## HOARDING/SAVING OBSESSIONS

(distinguish from hobbies and concern with objects of monetary or sentimental value)

_____ _____ –

## RELIGIOUS OBSESSIONS (scrupulosity)

| | | |
|---|---|---|
| _____ | _____ | Concerned with sacrilege and blasphemy |
| _____ | _____ | Excess concern with right/wrong, morality |
| _____ | _____ | Other_____ |

## OBSESSION WITH NEED FOR SYMMETRY OR EXACTNESS

| | | |
|---|---|---|
| _____ | _____ | Accompanied by magical thinking (e.g. concerned that mother will have accident unless things are in the right place) |
| _____ | _____ | Not accompanied by magical thinking |

## MISCELLANEOUS OBSESSIONS

| | | |
|---|---|---|
| _____ | _____ | Need to know or remember |
| _____ | _____ | Fear of saying certain things |
| _____ | _____ | Fear of not saying just the right thing |
| _____ | _____ | Fear of losing things |
| _____ | _____ | Intrusive (non-violent) images |
| _____ | _____ | Intrusive nonsense sounds, words, or music |
| _____ | _____ | Bothered by certain sounds/noises* |
| _____ | _____ | Lucky/unlucky numbers |
| _____ | _____ | Colours with special significance |
| _____ | _____ | Superstitious fears |
| _____ | _____ | Other_____ |

## SOMATIC OBSESSIONS

| | | |
|---|---|---|
| _____ | _____ | Concern with illness or disease* |
| _____ | _____ | Excessive concern with body part or aspect of appearance (e.g. dysmorphophobia)* |
| _____ | _____ | Other_____ |

CLEANING/WASHING COMPULSIONS

\_\_\_\_\_ \_\_\_\_\_ Excessive or ritualized handwashing

\_\_\_\_\_ \_\_\_\_\_ Excessive or ritualized showering, bathing, toothbrushing, grooming, or toilet routine

\_\_\_\_\_ \_\_\_\_\_ Involves cleaning of household items or other inanimate objects

\_\_\_\_\_ \_\_\_\_\_ Other measures to prevent or remove contact with contaminants

\_\_\_\_\_ \_\_\_\_\_ Other_____

CHECKING COMPULSIONS

\_\_\_\_\_ \_\_\_\_\_ Checking locks, stove, appliances, etc.

\_\_\_\_\_ \_\_\_\_\_ Checking that did not/will not harm others

\_\_\_\_\_ \_\_\_\_\_ Checking that did not/will not harm self

\_\_\_\_\_ \_\_\_\_\_ Checking that nothing terrible did/will happen

\_\_\_\_\_ \_\_\_\_\_ Checking that did not make mistake

\_\_\_\_\_ \_\_\_\_\_ Checking tied to somatic obsessions

\_\_\_\_\_ \_\_\_\_\_ Other_____

REPEATING RITUALS

\_\_\_\_\_ \_\_\_\_\_ Rereading or rewriting

\_\_\_\_\_ \_\_\_\_\_ Need to repeat routine activities (e.g. in/out door, up/down from chair)

\_\_\_\_\_ \_\_\_\_\_ Other_____

COUNTING COMPULSIONS

ORDERING/ARRANGING COMPULSIONS

HOARDING/COLLECTING COMPULSIONS

(distinguish from hobbies and concern with objects of monetary or sentimental value, e.g. carefully reads junk mail, piles up old newspapers, sorts through garbage, collects useless objects)

\_\_\_\_\_ \_\_\_\_\_ –

MISCELLANEOUS COMPULSIONS

\_\_\_\_\_ \_\_\_\_\_ Mental rituals (other than checking/counting)

\_\_\_\_\_ \_\_\_\_\_ Excessive list-making

\_\_\_\_\_ \_\_\_\_\_ Need to tell, ask, or confess

\_\_\_\_\_ \_\_\_\_\_ Need to touch, tap, or rub*

\_\_\_\_\_ \_\_\_\_\_ Rituals involving blinking or staring*

\_\_\_\_\_ \_\_\_\_\_ Measures (not checking) to prevent:

\_\_\_\_\_ \_\_\_\_\_ harm to self \_\_\_\_\_ ; harm to others \_\_\_\_\_ ; terrible

_____ _____ consequences _____

_____ _____ Ritualized eating behaviours*

_____ _____ Superstitious behaviours

_____ _____ Trichotillomania*

_____ _____ Other self-damaging or self-mutilating behaviours*

_____ _____ Other_____

# TARGET SYMPTOM LIST

Name_____ Date_____

OBSESSIONS:

1._____

_____

2._____

_____

3._____

_____

_____

COMPULSIONS:

1._____

_____

2._____

_____

3._____

_____

_____

AVOIDANCE:

1._____

_____

2._____

_____

3._____

_____

_____

# Y-BOCS SYMPTOM CHECKLIST (9/89)

## Y–BOCS severity ratings

### 1. Time occupied by obsessive thoughts

0 = None.

1 = Mild, <1 hr/day or occasional intrusion.

2 = Moderate, 1 to 3 hr/day or frequent intrusion.

3 = Severe, >3 and up to 8 hr/day or very frequent intrusion.

4 = Extreme, >8 hr/day or near constant intrusion.

### 1b. Obsession-free interval (not included in total score)

0 = No symptoms.

1 = Long symptom-free interval, >8 consecutive hr/day symptom-free.

2 = Moderately long symptom-free interval, >3 and up to 8 consecutive hr/day symptom-free.

3 = Short symptom-free interval, from 1 to 3 consecutive hr/day symptom-free.

4 = Extremely short symptom-free interval, <1 consecutive hr/day symptom-free.

### 2. Interference due to obsessive thoughts

0 = None.

1 = Mild, slight interference with social or occupational activities, but overall performance not impaired.

2 = Moderate, definite interference with social or occupational performance, but still manageable.

3 = Severe, causes substantial impairment in social or occupational performance.

4 = Extreme, incapacitating.

### 3. Distress associated with obsessive thoughts

0 = None.

1 = Mild, not too disturbing.

2 = Moderate, disturbing, but still manageable.

3 = Severe, very disturbing.

4 = Extreme, near constant and disabling distress.

### 4. Resistance against obsessions

0 = Makes an effort always to resist, or symptoms so minimal doesn't need actively to resist.

1 = Tries to resist most of the time.

2 = Makes some effort to resist.

3 = Yields to all obsessions without attempting to control them, but does so with some reluctance.

4 = Completely and willingly yields to all obsessions.

### 5. Degree of control over obsessive thoughts

0 = Complete control.

Reproduced from *Arch. Gen. Psych.*, **46**(11), Goodman, W.K., Price, L.H., Rasmussen, S.A., et al., The Yale Brown Obsessive Compulsive Scale. I. Development, use and reliability, p. 1006 -11, Copyright (1989), with permission from the American Medical Association

1 = Much control, usually able to stop or divert obsessions with some effort and concentration.

2 = Moderate control, sometimes able to stop or divert obsessions.

3 = Little control, rarely successful in stopping or dismissing obsessions, can only divert attention with difficulty.

4 = No control, experienced as completely involuntary, rarely able, even momentarily, to alter obsessive thinking.

### 6. Time spent performing compulsive behaviours

0 = None.

1 = Mild (spends <1 hr/day performing compulsions), or occasional performance of compulsive behaviours.

2 = Moderate (spends from 1 to 3 hr/day performing compulsions), or frequent performance of compulsive behaviours.

3 = Severe (spends >3 and up to 8 hr/day performing compulsions), or very frequent performance of compulsive behaviours.

4 = Extreme (spends >8 hr/day performing compulsions), or near constant performance of compulsive behaviours (too numerous to count).

### 6b. Compulsion-free interval (not included in total score)

0 = No symptoms.

1 = Long symptom-free interval, >8 consecutive hr/day symptom-free.

2 = Moderately long symptom-free interval, >3 and up to 8 consecutive hr/day symptom-free.

3 = Short symptom-free interval, from 1 to 3 consecutive hr/day symptom-free.

4 = Extremely short symptom-free interval, <1 consecutive hr/day symptom-free.

### 7. Interference due to compulsive behaviours

0 = None.

1 = Mild, slight interference with social or occupational activities, but overall performance not impaired.

2 = Moderate, definite interference with social or occupational performance, but still manageable.

3 = Severe, causes substantial impairment in social or occupational performance.

4 = Extreme, incapacitating.

### 8. Distress associated with compulsive behaviour

0 = None.

1 = Mild, only slightly anxious if compulsions prevented, or only slight anxiety during performance of compulsions.

2 = Moderate, reports that anxiety would mount but remain manageable if compulsions prevented, or that anxiety increases but remains manageable during performance of compulsions.

3 = Severe, prominent and very disturbing increase in anxiety if compulsions interrupted, or prominent and very disturbing increase in anxiety during performance of compulsions.

4 = Extreme, incapacitating anxiety from any intervention aimed at modifying activity, or incapacitating anxiety develops during performance of compulsions.

### 9. Resistance against compulsions

0 = Makes an effort to always resist, or symptoms so minimal doesn't need actively to resist.

1 = Tries to resist most of the time.

2 = Makes some effort to resist.

3 = Yields to almost all compulsions without attempting to control them but does so with some reluctance.

4 = Completely and willingly yields to all compulsions.

### 10. Degree of control over compulsive behaviour

0 = Complete control.

1 = Much control, experiences pressure to perform the behaviour but usually able to exercise voluntary control over it.

2 = Moderate control, strong pressure to perform behaviour, can control it only with difficulty.

3 = Little control, very strong drive to perform behaviour, must be carried to completion, can only delay with difficulty.

4 = No control, drive to perform behaviour experienced as completely involuntary and overpowering, rarely able even momentarily to delay activity.

('The remaining questions are about both obsessions and compulsions. Some ask about related problems.' These are investigational items not included in total Y-BOCS score but may be useful in assessing these symptoms.)

### 11. Insight into obsessions and compulsions

0 = Excellent insight, fully rational.

1 = Good insight. Readily acknowledges absurdity or excessiveness of thoughts or behaviours but does not seem completely convinced that there isn't something besides anxiety to be concerned about (i.e. has lingering doubts).

2 = Fair insight. Reluctantly admits thoughts or behaviour seem unreasonable or excessive, but wavers. May have some unrealistic fears, but no fixed convictions.

3 = Poor insight. Maintains that thoughts or behaviours are not unreasonable or excessive, but acknowledges validity of contrary evidence (i.e. overvalued ideas present).

4 = Lacks insight, delusional. Definitely convinced that concerns and behaviour are reasonable, unresponsive to contrary evidence.

### 12. Avoidance

0 = No deliberate avoidance.

1 = Mild, minimal avoidance.

2 = Moderate, some avoidance; clearly present.

3 = Severe, much avoidance; avoidance prominent.

4 = Extreme, very extensive avoidance; patient does almost everything he/she can to avoid triggering symptoms.

### 13. Degree of indecisiveness

0 = None.

1 = Mild, some trouble in making decisions about minor things.

2 = Moderate, freely reports significant trouble in making decisions that others would not think twice about.

3 = Severe, continual weighing of pros and cons about non-essentials.

4 = Extreme, unable to make any decisions. Disabling.

### 14. Overvalued sense of responsibility

0 = None.

1 = Mild, only mentioned on questioning, slight sense of over-responsibility.

2 = Moderate, ideas stated spontaneously, clearly present; patient experiences significant sense of over-responsibility for events outside his/her reasonable control.

3 = Severe, ideas prominent and pervasive; deeply concerned he/she is responsible for events clearly outside his control. Self-blaming far-fetched and nearly irrational.

4 = Extreme, delusional sense of responsibility (e.g. if an earthquake occurs 3000 miles away, patient blames herself because she didn't perform her compulsions).

### 15. Pervasive slowness/disturbance of inertia

0 = None.

1 = Mild, occasional delay in starting or finishing.

2 = Moderate, frequent prolongation of routine activities, but tasks usually completed. Frequently late.

3 = Severe, pervasive and marked difficulty initiating and completing routine tasks. Usually late.

4 = Extreme, unable to start or complete routine tasks without full assistance.

### 16. Pathological doubting

0 = None.

1 = Mild, only mentioned on questioning, slight pathological doubt. Examples given may be within normal range.

2 = Moderate, ideas stated spontaneously, clearly present and apparent in some of patient's behaviours; patient bothered by significant pathological doubt. Some effect on performance, but still manageable.

3 = Severe, uncertainty about perceptions or memory prominent; pathological doubt frequently affects performance.

4 = Extreme, uncertainty about perceptions constantly present; pathological doubt substantially affects almost all activities. Incapacitating (e.g. patient states 'my mind doesn't trust what my eyes see').

(Items 17 and 18 refer to global illness severity. The rater is required to consider global function, not just the severity of obsessive–compulsive symptoms.)

### 17. Global severity: Interviewer's judgement of the overall severity of the patient's illness

0 = No illness.

1 = Illness slight, doubtful, transient; no functional impairment.

2 = Mild symptoms, little functional impairment.

3 = Moderate symptoms, functions with effort.

4 = Moderate–severe symptoms, limited functioning.

5 = Severe symptoms, functions mainly with assistance.

6 = Extremely severe symptoms, completely non-functional.

18. **Global improvement: Interviewer's judgement of the total overall improvement present since the initial rating whether or not, in your judgement, it is due to drug treatment**

0 = Very much worse.

1 = Much worse.

2 = Minimally worse.

3 = No change.

4 = Minimally improved.

5 = Much improved.

6 = Very much improved.

19. **Reliability: Interviewer's judgement of the overall reliability of the rating scores** obtained.

0 = Excellent, no reason to suspect data unreliable.

1 = Good, factor(s) present that may adversely affect reliability.

2 = Fair, factor(s) present that definitely reduce reliability.

3 = Poor, very low reliability.

Items 17 and 18 are adapted from the Clinical Global Impression Scale (Guy, W. (1976) *ECDEU Assessment Manual for Psychopharmacology: Publication 76–338*. US Department of Health, Education, and Welfare, Washington, D.C.).

## Yale–Brown Obsessive Compulsive Scale (9/89)

**Y-BOCS TOTAL (add items 1–10)**

Patient name _____     Date _____

Patient ID _____     Rater _____

| | | None | Mild | Moderate | Severe | Extreme |
|---|---|---|---|---|---|---|
| 1. | Time spent on obsessions | 0 | 1 | 2 | 3 | 4 |

| 1b. | Obsession-free interval | | | | | |
|---|---|---|---|---|---|---|
| | | No symptoms | Long | Moderately long | Short | Extremely short |
| | (do not add to subtotal or total score) | 0 | 1 | 2 | 3 | 4 |

| | | None | Mild | Moderate | Severe | Extreme |
|---|---|---|---|---|---|---|
| 2. | Interference from obsessions | 0 | 1 | 2 | 3 | 4 |
| 3. | Distress of obsessions | 0 | 1 | 2 | 3 | 4 |

| | | Always resists | | | | Completely yields |
|---|---|---|---|---|---|---|
| 4. | Resistance | 0 | 1 | 2 | 3 | 4 |

| | | Complete control | Much control | Moderate control | Little control | No control |
|---|---|---|---|---|---|---|
| 5. | Control over obsessions | 0 | 1 | 2 | 3 | 4 |

**OBSESSION SUBTOTAL (add items 1–5)**

| | | None | Mild | Moderate | Severe | Extreme |
|---|---|---|---|---|---|---|
| 6. | Time spent on compulsions | 0 | 1 | 2 | 3 | 4 |

| 6b. | Compulsion-free interval | | | | | |
|---|---|---|---|---|---|---|
| | | No symptoms | Long | Moderately long | Short | Extremely short |
| | (do not add to subtotal or total score | 0 | 1 | 2 | 3 | 4 |

| | | None | Mild | Moderate | Severe | Extreme |
|---|---|---|---|---|---|---|
| 7. | Interference from compulsions | 0 | 1 | 2 | 3 | 4 |

Reproduced from *Arch. Gen. Psych.*, **46**(11), Goodman, W.K., Price, L.H., Rasmussen, S.A., et al., The Yale Brown Obsessive Compulsive Scale. I. Development, use and reliability, p. 1006 –11, Copyright (1989), with permission from the American Medical Association

| 8. | Distress from compulsions | 0 | 1 | 2 | 3 | 4 |
|----|----|----|----|----|----|----|
|    |    | Always resists | | Completely yields | | |
| 9. | Resistance | 0 | 1 | 2 | 3 | 4 |
|    |    | Complete control | Much control | Moderate control | Little control | No control |
| 10. | Control over compulsions | 0 | 1 | 2 | 3 | 4 |

COMPULSION SUBTOTAL (add items 6–10)

|    |    | Excellent | | | | Absent |
|----|----|----|----|----|----|----|
| 11. | Insight into O-C symptoms | 0 | 1 | 2 | 3 | 4 |
|    |    | None | Mild | Moderate | Severe | Extreme |
| 12. | Avoidance | 0 | 1 | 2 | 3 | 4 |
| 13. | Indecisiveness | 0 | 1 | 2 | 3 | 4 |
| 14. | Pathological responsibility | 0 | 1 | 2 | 3 | 4 |
| 15. | Slowness | 0 | 1 | 2 | 3 | 4 |
| 16. | Pathological doubting | 0 | 1 | 2 | 3 | 4 |
| 17. | Global severity | 0 | 1 | 2 | 3 | 4 | 5 | 6 |
| 18. | Global improvement | 0 | 1 | 2 | 3 | 4 | 5 | 6 |
| 19. | Reliability | Excellent = 0 | Good = 1 | Fair = 2 | Poor = 3 |

# Children's Yale–Brown Obsessive Compulsive Scale (CY-BOCS)

The Children's Yale–Brown Obsessive Compulsive Scale (CY-BOCS) is a commonly used clinician-rated scale of paediatric obsessive–compulsive symptom severity. It is a modified version of the original Y-BOCS scale (Goodman et al. 1989).

## Reference

Goodman WK, et al. (1989). The Yale-Brown Obsessive Compulsive Scale. I. Development, use and reliability. *Arch Gen Psych*. 46: 1006–11.

## CY-BOCS obsessions checklist

| (1) | X | Contamination obsessions | Current | Past | Trauma-related | Non-trauma-related |
|---|---|---|---|---|---|---|
| | | Concern with dirt, germs, certain illnesses (e.g. AIDS) | | | | |
| | | Concern or disgust with bodily waste or secretions (e.g. urine, faeces, saliva) | | | | |
| | | Excessive concern with environmental contaminants (e.g. asbestos, radiation, toxic waste) | | | | |
| | | Excessive concern with household items (e.g. cleaners, solvents) | | | | |
| | | Excessively bothered by sticky substances or residues | | | | |
| | | Concerned will get ill because of contaminant | | | | |
| | | Concerned will get others ill by spreading contaminant | | | | |
| | | No concern with consequences of contamination other than how it might feel* | | | | |

| (2) | X | Aggressive obsessions | Current | Past | Trauma-related | Non-trauma-related |
|---|---|---|---|---|---|---|
| | | Fear might harm self | | | | |
| | | Fear might harm others | | | | |
| | | Fear harm will come to self | | | | |
| | | Fear harm will come to others (may be because of something child did or did not do) | | | | |
| | | Violent or horrific images | | | | |
| | | Fear of blurting out obscenities or insults | | | | |
| | | Fear of doing something else embarrassing* | | | | |
| | | Fear will act on unwanted impulses (e.g. to stab a family member) | | | | |
| | | Fear will steal things | | | | |

Fear will be responsible for
something else terrible happening (e.g. fire, burglary,
flood)

| (3) | X | **Sexual obsessions** | **Current** | **Past** | **Trauma-related** | **Non-trauma-related** |
|---|---|---|---|---|---|---|

Ask the child, 'Are you
having any sexual thoughts?'
If yes,

'Are they routine or are
they repetitive thoughts
that you would rather not
have or find disturbing?'
If yes,

'Are they … forbidden or
perverse sexual thoughts,
images, or impulses?'

Content involves
homosexuality

Sexual behaviour towards
others (aggressive)

| (4) | X | **Hoarding/saving obsessions** | **Current** | **Past** | **Trauma-related** | **Non-trauma-related** |
|---|---|---|---|---|---|---|

Fear of losing things

| (5) | X | **Magical thoughts/super-stitious obsessions** | **Current** | **Past** | **Trauma-related** | **Non-trauma-related** |
|---|---|---|---|---|---|---|

Lucky/unlucky numbers, col-
ours, words

| (6) | X | **Somatic obsessions** | **Current** | **Past** | **Trauma-related** | **Non-trauma-related** |
|---|---|---|---|---|---|---|

Excessive concern with illness
or disease*

Excessive concern with body
part or aspect of appearance
(e.g. dysmorphophobia)

| (7) | X | **Religious obsessions** | **Current** | **Past** | **Trauma-related** | **Non-trauma-related** |
|---|---|---|---|---|---|---|

Excessive concern or fear of
offending religious objects
(God)

Excessive concern with right/
wrong, morality

| (8) X Miscellaneous obsessions | Current | Past | Trauma-related | Non-trauma-related |
|---|---|---|---|---|
| The need to know or remember | | | | |
| Fear of saying certain things | | | | |
| Fear of not saying just the right thing | | | | |
| Intrusive (non-violent) images | | | | |
| Intrusive sounds, words, music, or numbers | | | | |

**Target symptom list for obsessions**

| Please list the obsessions experienced. Note if absent. | Trauma-related | Non-trauma-related |
|---|---|---|
| 1. | | |
| 2. | | |
| 3. | | |
| 4. | | |

## CY-BOCS compulsions checklist

Check all symptoms that apply.

| Washing/cleaning compulsions | Current | Past | TR | NTR |
|---|---|---|---|---|
| Excessive or ritualized handwashing | | | | |
| Excessive or ritualized showering, bathing, tooth-brushing, grooming, toilet routine | | | | |
| Excessive cleaning of items (such as personal clothes or important objects) | | | | |
| Other measures to prevent or remove contact with contaminants | | | | |
| Other (describe) | | | | |

| Checking compulsions | Current | Past | TR | NTR |
|---|---|---|---|---|
| Checking locks, toys, school books/items, etc. | | | | |
| Checking associated with getting washed, dressed, or undressed | | | | |
| Checking that did not/will not harm others | | | | |
| Checking that did not/will not harm self | | | | |
| Checking that nothing terrible did/will happen | | | | |
| Checking that did not make a mistake | | | | |
| Checking tied to somatic obsessions | | | | |
| Other | | | | |

| Repeating rituals | Current | Past | TR | NTR |
|---|---|---|---|---|
| Rereading, erasing, or rewriting | | | | |
| Need to repeat routine activities (e.g. in/out of doorway, up/down from chair) | | | | |
| Other | | | | |

| Counting compulsions | Current | Past | TR | NTR |
|---|---|---|---|---|
| Objects, certain numbers, words, etc. | | | | |
| Other | | | | |

| Ordering/arranging | Current | Past | TR | NTR |
|---|---|---|---|---|
| Need for symmetry/evening up (e.g. lining items up a certain way or arranging personal items in specific patterns) | | | | |
| Other | | | | |

| Hoarding/saving compulsions | Current | Past | TR | NTR |
|---|---|---|---|---|
| Distinguish from hobbies and concern with objects of monetary or sentimental value | | | | |
| Difficulty throwing things away, saving bits of paper, string, etc. | | | | |
| Other | | | | |

| Excessive games/superstitious behaviours | Current | Past | TR | NTR |
|---|---|---|---|---|
| Distinguish from age-appropriate magical games (e.g. array of behaviour, such as stepping over certain spots on a floor, touching an object/self certain number of times as a routine game to avoid something bad from happening) | | | | |
| Other | | | | |

| Rituals involving other persons | Current | Past | TR | NTR |
|---|---|---|---|---|
| The need to involve another person (usually a parent) in ritual (e.g. asking a parent to repeatedly answer the same question, making mother perform certain mealtime rituals involving specific utensils) | | | | |
| Other (describe) | | | | |

| Miscellaneous compulsions | Current | Past | TR | NTR |
|---|---|---|---|---|
| Mental rituals (other than checking/counting) | | | | |
| The need to tell, ask, or confess | | | | |
| Measures (not checking) to prevent harm to self, harm to others, or terrible consequences | | | | |
| Ritualized eating behaviours* | | | | |
| Excessive list-making* | | | | |
| Need to touch, tap, rub* | | | | |
| Need to do things (e.g. touch or arrange) until it feels just right* | | | | |
| Rituals involving blinking or staring* | | | | |
| Trichotillomania (hair-pulling)* | | | | |
| Other self-damaging or self-mutilating behaviours | | | | |
| Other | | | | |

| Target symptom list for compulsions | | | |
|---|---|---|---|
| Please list the compulsions experienced. Note if absent. | | TR | NTR |
| 1. | | | |
| 2. | | | |
| 3. | | | |
| 4. | | | |

1.  Are the obsessions part of the principal/target symptoms?

| Yes | No |
|-----|-----|

2.  Are the compulsions part of the principal/target symptoms?

| Yes | No |
|-----|-----|

3.  When did the trauma-related obsessions begin?

_____

_____

4.  When did the non-trauma-related obsessions begin?

_____

_____

5.  When did the trauma-related compulsions begin?

_____

_____

6.  When did the non-trauma-related compulsions begin?

_____

_____

## CY-BOCS severity ratings

1. *Time occupied by obsessive thoughts*

    0 = **None**.

    1 = **Mild**, <1 hr/day or occasional intrusion.

    2 = **Moderate**, 1–3 hr/day or frequent intrusion.

    3 = **Severe**, >3 and up to 8 hr/day or very frequent intrusion.

    4 = **Extreme**, >8 hr/day or near constant intrusion.

1B. *Obsession-free interval (not included in total score)*

    0 = **None**.

    1 = **Mild**, long symptom-free intervals, >8 consecutive hr/day symptom-free.

    2 = **Moderate**, moderately long symptom-free intervals, >3 and up to 8 consecutive hr/day symptom-free.

    3 = **Severe**, brief symptom-free intervals, from 1 to 3 consecutive hr/day symptom-free.

    4 = **Extreme**, <1 consecutive hr/day symptom-free.

2. *Interference due to obsessive thoughts*

    0 = **None**.

    1 = **Mild**, slight interference with social or school activities, but overall performance not impaired.

    2 = **Moderate**, definite interference with social or school performance, but still manageable.

    3 = **Severe**, causes substantial impairment in social or school performance.

    4 = **Extreme**, incapacitating.

3. *Distress associated with obsessive thoughts*

    0 = **None**.

    1 = **Mild**, infrequent and not too disturbing.

    2 = **Moderate**, frequent and disturbing, but still manageable.

    3 = **Severe**, very frequent and very disturbing.

    4 = **Extreme**, near constant and disabling distress/frustration.

4. *Resistance against obsessions*

    0 = **None**, makes an effort always to resist, or symptoms so minimal doesn't need to actively resist.

    1 = **Mild**, tries to resist most of the time.

    2 = **Moderate**, makes some effort to resist.

    3 = **Severe**, yields to all obsessions without attempting to control them, but does so with some reluctance.

    4 = **Extreme**, completely and willingly yields to all obsessions.

5. *Degree of control over obsessive thoughts*

    0 = **Complete control**.

    1 = **Much control**, usually able to stop or divert obsessions with some effort and concentration.

    2 = **Moderate control**, sometimes able to stop or divert obsessions.

3 = **Little control**, rarely successful in stopping obsessions, can only divert attention with difficulty.

4 = **No control**, experienced as completely involuntary, rarely able, even momentarily, to divert thinking.

## Questions on compulsions (items 6–10)

### 6A. Time spent performing compulsive behaviours

0 = **None**.

1 = **Mild**, spends <1 hr/day performing compulsions, or occasional performance of compulsive behaviours.

2 = **Moderate**, spends from 1 to 3 hr/day performing compulsions, or frequent performance of compulsions.

3 = **Severe**, spends >3 and up to 8 hr/day performing compulsions, or very frequent performance of compulsions.

4 = **Extreme**, spends >8 hr/day performing compulsions, or near constant performance of compulsive behaviours (too numerous to count).

### 6B. Compulsion-free interval

0 = **No symptoms**.

1 = **Mild**, long symptom-free interval, >8 consecutive hr/day symptom-free.

2 = **Moderate**, moderately long symptom-free interval, >3 and up to 8 consecutive hr/day symptom-free.

3 = **Severe**, short symptom-free interval, from 1 to 3 consecutive hr/day symptom-free.

4 = **Extreme**, <1 consecutive hr/day symptom-free.

### 7. Interference due to compulsive behaviours

0 = **None**.

1 = **Mild**, slight interference with social or school activities, but overall performance not impaired.

2 = **Moderate**, definite interference with social or school performance, but still manageable.

3 = **Severe**, causes substantial impairment in social or school performance.

4 = **Extreme**, incapacitating.

### 8. Distress associated with compulsive behaviour

0 = **None**.

1 = **Mild**, only slightly anxious/frustrated if compulsions prevented, or only slight anxiety/frustration during performance of compulsions.

2 = **Moderate**, reports that anxiety/frustration would mount but remain manageable if compulsions prevented. Anxiety/frustration increases but remains manageable during performance of compulsions.

3 = **Severe**, prominent and very disturbing increase in anxiety/frustration if compulsions interrupted. Prominent and very disturbing increase in anxiety/frustration during performance of compulsions.

4 = **Extreme**, Incapacitating anxiety/frustration from any intervention aimed at modifying activity. Incapacitating anxiety/frustration develops during performance of compulsions.

**9. Resistance against compulsions**

0 = **None**, makes an effort always to resist, or symptoms so minimal doesn't need to actively resist.

1 = **Mild**, tries to resist most of the time.

2 = **Moderate**, makes some effort to resist.

3 = **Severe**, yields to almost all compulsions without attempting to control them but does so with some reluctance.

4 = **Extreme**, completely and willingly yields to all compulsions.

**10. Degree of control over compulsive behaviour**

0 = **Complete control**.

1 = **Much control**, experiences pressure to perform the behaviour but usually able to exercise voluntary control over it.

2 = **Moderate control**, moderate control, strong pressure to perform behaviour, can control it only with difficulty.

3 = **Little control**, little control, very strong drive to perform behaviour, must be carried to completion, can only delay with difficulty.

4 = **No control**, no control, drive to perform behaviour experienced as completely involuntary and overpowering, rarely able to delay activity (even momentarily).

**11. Insight into obsessions and compulsions**

0 = **None**, excellent insight, fully rational.

1 = **Mild**, good insight, readily acknowledges absurdity or excessiveness of thoughts or behaviours but does not seem completely convinced that there isn't something besides anxiety to be concerned about (i.e. has lingering doubts).

2 = **Moderate**, fair insight, reluctantly admits thoughts or behaviour seem unreasonable or excessive but wavers. May have some unrealistic fears, but no fixed convictions.

3 = **Severe**, poor insight, maintains that thoughts or behaviours are not reasonable or excessive but wavers. May have some unrealistic fears but acknowledges validity of contrary evidence (i.e. overvalued ideas present).

4 = **Extreme**, lacks insight, delusional, definitely convinced that concerns and behaviour are reasonable, unresponsive to contrary evidence.

**12. Avoidance**

0 = **None**.

1 = **Mild**, minimal avoidance.

2 = **Moderate**, some avoidance; clearly present.

3 = **Severe**, much avoidance; avoidance prominent.

4 = **Extreme**, very extensive avoidance; patient does almost everything he/she can to avoid triggering symptoms.

**13. Degree of indecisiveness**

0 = **None**.

1 = **Mild**, some trouble making decisions about minor things.

2 = **Moderate**, freely reports significant trouble in making decisions that others would not think twice about.

3 = **Severe**, continual weighing of pros and cons about non-essentials.

4 = **Extreme**, unable to make any decisions, disabling.

### 14. Overvalued sense of responsibility

0 = **None**.

1 = **Mild**, only mentioned on questioning, slight sense of over-responsibility.

2 = **Moderate**, ideas stated spontaneously, clearly present; patient experiences significant sense of over-responsibility for events outside his/her reasonable control.

3 = **Severe**, ideas prominent and pervasive; deeply concerned he/she is responsible for events clearly outside his control, self-blaming far-fetched and nearly irrational.

4 = **Extreme**, Delusional sense of responsibility (e.g. if an earthquake occurs 3000 miles away, patient blames himself because he didn't perform his compulsion).

### 15. Pervasive slowness/disturbance of inertia

0 = **None**.

1 = **Mild**, occasional delay in starting or finishing tasks/activities.

2 = **Moderate**, frequent prolongation of routine activities, but tasks usually completed, frequently late.

3 = **Severe**, pervasive and marked difficulty initiating and completing routine tasks, usually late.

4 = **Extreme**, unable to start or complete routine tasks without full assistance.

### 16. Pathological doubting

0 = **None**.

1 = **Mild**, only mentioned on questioning, slight pathological doubt, examples given may be within normal range.

2 = **Moderate**, ideas stated spontaneously, clearly present and apparent in some of patient's behaviours; patient bothered by significant pathological doubt. Some effect on performance, but still manageable.

3 = **Severe**, uncertainty about perceptions or memory prominent; pathological doubt frequently affects performance.

4 = **Extreme**, uncertainty about perceptions constantly present; pathological doubt substantially affects almost all activities, incapacitating (e.g. patient states 'my mind doesn't trust what my eyes see').

### 17. Global severity

Interviewer's judgement of the overall severity of the patient's illness. Rated from 0 (no illness) to 6 (most severe patient seen). (Consider the degree of distress reported by the patient, the symptoms observed, and the functional impairment reported. Your judgement is required both in averaging these data as well as weighing the reliability or accuracy of the data obtained.)

0 = **No illness**.

1 = **Slight**, illness slight, doubtful, transient; no functional impairment.

2 = **Mild**, little functional impairment.

3 = **Moderate**, functions with effort.

4 = **Moderate–severe**, limited functioning.

5 = **Severe**, functions mainly with assistance.

6 = **Extremely severe**, completely non-functional.

### 18. *Global improvement*

Rate total overall improvement present since the initial rating whether or not, in your judgement, it is due to treatment.

0 = **Very much worse**.

1 = **Much worse**.

2 = **Minimally worse**.

3 = **No change**.

4 = **Minimally improved**.

5 = **Much improved**.

6 = **Very much improved**.

### 19. *Reliability*

Rate the overall reliability of the rating scores obtained. Factors that may affect reliability include the patient's cooperativeness and his/her natural ability to communicate. The type and severity of obsessive–compulsive symptoms present may interfere with the patient's concentration, attention, or freedom to speak spontaneously (e.g. the content of some obsessions may cause the patient to choose his words very carefully).

0 = **Excellent**, no reason to suspect data unreliable.

1 = **Good**, factor(s) present that may adversely affect reliability.

2 = **Fair**, factor(s) present that definitely reduce reliability.

3 = **Poor**, very low reliability.

### Children's Yale–Brown Obsessive Compulsive Scale

**CY-BOCS TOTAL (add items 1–10)**

Patient name _____  Date _____

Patient ID _____  Rater _____

|  |  | **None** | **Mild** | **Moderate** | **Severe** | **Extreme** |
|---|---|---|---|---|---|---|
| 1. | Time spent on obsessions | 0 | 1 | 2 | 3 | 4 |
|  |  | No symptoms | Long | Moderately long | Short | Extremely short |
| 1b. | Obsession-free interval (do not add to subtotal or total score) | 0 | 1 | 2 | 3 | 4 |
| 2. | Interference from obsessions | 0 | 1 | 2 | 3 | 4 |
| 3. | Distress of obsessions | 0 | 1 | 2 | 3 | 4 |
|  |  | Always resists |  |  |  | Completely yields |
| 4. | Resistance | 0 | 1 | 2 | 3 | 4 |
|  |  | Complete control | Much control | Moderate control | Little control | No control |
| 5. | Control over obsessions | 0 | 1 | 2 | 3 | 4 |
|  | OBSESSION SUBTOTAL (add items 1–5) |  |  |  | TR | NTR |

|  |  | **None** | **Mild** | **Moderate** | **Severe** | **Extreme** |
|---|---|---|---|---|---|---|
| 6. | Time spent on compulsions | 0 | 1 | 2 | 3 | 4 |
|  |  | No symptoms | Long | Moderately long | Short | Extremely short |
| 6b. | Compulsion-free interval (do not add to subtotal or total score) | 0 | 1 | 2 | 3 | 4 |
| 7. | Interference from compulsions | 0 | 1 | 2 | 3 | 4 |
| 8. | Distress from compulsions | 0 | 1 | 2 | 3 | 4 |
|  |  | Always resists |  |  |  | Completely yields |
| 9. | Resistance | 0 | 1 | 2 | 3 | 4 |
|  |  | Complete control | Much control | Moderate control | Little control | No control |
| 10. | Control over compulsions | 0 | 1 | 2 | 3 | 4 |
|  | COMPULSION SUBTOTAL (add items 6–10) |  |  |  | TR | NTR |
|  |  | Excellent |  |  |  | Absent |
| 11. | Insight into O-C symptoms | 0 | 1 | 2 | 3 | 4 |

|  | None | Mild | Moderate | Severe | Extreme |
|---|---|---|---|---|---|
| 12. Avoidance | 0 | 1 | 2 | 3 | 4 |
| 13. Indecisiveness | 0 | 1 | 2 | 3 | 4 |
| 14. Pathological responsibility | 0 | 1 | 2 | 3 | 4 |
| 15. Slowness | 0 | 1 | 2 | 3 | 4 |
| 16. Pathological doubting | 0 | 1 | 2 | 3 | 4 |
| 17. Global severity | 0 1 | 2 | 3 | 4 | 5 | 6 |
| 18. Global improvement | 0 1 | 2 | 3 | 4 | 5 | 6 |
| 19. Reliability | Excellent = 0 | Good = 1 | Fair = 2 | Poor = 3 |

Reproduced from *Arch. Gen. Psych.*, **46**(11), Goodman, W.K., Price, L.H., Rasmussen, S.A., *et al.*, The Yale Brown Obsessive Compulsive Scale. I. Development, use and reliability, p. 1006–11, Copyright (1989), with permission from the American Medical Association.

## Appendix 4

# Dimensional Yale–Brown Obsessive Compulsive Severity Scale (DY-BOCS)

The Dimensional Yale–Brown Obsessive Compulsive Scale (DY-BOCS) is an extension of the original Yale–Brown Obsessive Compulsive Scale (Y-BOCS) that is designed to evaluate the nature and current severity of obsessive–compulsive symptoms. DY-BOCS includes specific symptom checklists/severity ratings for the following symptom categories: (1) aggressive obsessions and related compulsions; (2) sexual and religious obsessions and related compulsions; (3) symmetry, ordering, counting, and arranging obsessions and compulsions; (4) contamination obsessions and cleaning compulsions; (5) hoarding and collecting obsessions and compulsions; (6) somatic obsessions and compulsions; and (7) miscellaneous symptoms.

## References

Goodman WK, et al. (1989). The Yale-Brown Obsessive Compulsive Scale. I. Development, use and reliability. Arch Gen Psychiatry. **46**: 1006–11.

Leckman JF, et al. (1997). Symptoms of obsessive–compulsive disorder. Am J Psychiatry. **154**: 911–17.

Mataix-Cols D, et al. (1999). Use of factor-analyzed symptom dimensions to predict outcome with serotonin reuptake inhibitors and placebo in the treatment of obsessive–compulsive disorder. Am J Psychiatry. **156**: 1409–16.

Summerfeldt L.J, et al. (1999). Symptom structure in obsessive–compulsive disorder: a confirmatory factor-analytic study. Behav Res Ther. **37**: 297–311.

Clinicians interested in using this scale and/or obtaining the full instructions should contact Dr James Leckman at Child Study Center, Yale University School of Medicine, New Haven, CT 06520-7900, USA.

## Checklist of aggressive obsessions and related compulsions (past week)

**Checklist**: check once (✓) for any symptoms present during the past week.

Here the emphasis is on aggressive thoughts and images. Care may be needed to distinguish between contamination and somatic obsessions. The term 'harm' was used in the self-report. It is inherently ambiguous, and some subjects may have checked some of the harm items when the symptoms are best understood in another context, i.e. contamination or somatic worries. Check only if clear that obsessions or compulsions are present and have aggressive content.

| *Aggressive obsessions* | *Related compulsions* |
|---|---|
| ___ Might harm self (aggressive content) | ___ Checking that no harm to self has occurred |
| ___ Might be harmed (aggressive content) | |
| ___ Might harm loved ones unintentionally (close family members) | |
| ___ Might harm others unintentionally | ___ Checking that no harm to others |
| ___ Might harm loved ones intentionally has occurred (close family members) | |
| ___ Might harm others intentionally | ___ Checking compulsions to prevent harm |
| ___ Might be responsible for something else terrible happening | |
| ___ Violent or horrific images | ___ Repeating to prevent harm |
| ___ Might blurt out obscenities or insults | ___ Mental rituals to prevent harm |
| ___ Might do something embarrassing | |
| ___ Might be responsible for something terrible | ___ Checking that nothing terrible has happened |
| ___ Might act on other unwanted aggressive impulses | |
| ___ Might say harmful things (aggressive content) | |

### Avoidance—aggressive obsessions
___ Intentional avoidance of people, places, or things because of any of the above obsessions or compulsions concerning aggressive obsessions

### Other obsessions or compulsions in this category (describe):

_____

_____

### Symptoms in this category were present during the past week?
Yes    No

If yes, complete the next page. If no, skip to next section.

## Severity ratings (past week) for aggressive obsessions and related compulsions

*1. How much of your time is occupied by these obsessions and compulsions?*

0 = **No time at all**.

1 = **Rarely**, present during the past week, often not on a daily basis, typically <3 hr/week.

2 = **Occasionally, >3 hr/week, but <1 hr/day**—occasional intrusion, need to perform compulsions, or avoidance (occurs no >5 times a day).

3 = **Frequently, 1 to 3 hr/day**—frequent intrusion, need to perform compulsions, or avoidance (occurs >8 times a day, but most hours of the day are free of these obsessions, compulsions, and related avoidance).

4 = **Almost always, >3 and up to 8 hr/day**—very frequent intrusion, need to perform compulsions, or avoidance (occurs >8 times a day and occurs during most hours of the day).

5 = **Always, >8 hr/day**—near constant intrusion of obsessions, need to perform compulsions, or avoidance (too numerous to count, and an hour rarely passes without several obsessions, compulsions, and/or avoidance).

*2. How much distress do these obsessions and related compulsions cause?*

0 = **No distress**.

1 = **Minimal**, when symptoms are present they are minimally distressing.

2 = **Mild**, some clear distress present, but not too disturbing.

3 = **Moderate**, disturbing, but still tolerable.

4 = **Severe**, very disturbing.

5 = **Extreme**, near constant and disabling distress.

*3. How much do these obsessions and related compulsions interfere with your family life, friendships, or ability to perform well at work or at school?*

0 = **No interference**.

1 = **Minimal**, slight interference with social or occupational activities, overall performance not impaired.

2 = **Mild**, some interference with social or occupational activities, overall performance affected to a small degree.

3 = **Moderate**, definite interference with social or occupational performance, but still manageable.

4 = **Severe interference**, causes substantial impairment in social or occupational performance.

5 = **Extreme**, incapacitating interference.

Reproduced with permission from Dr James Leckman.

## Checklist of sexual and religious obsessions and related compulsions severity ratings (past week)

*Checklist:* check once (✓) for any symptoms present during the past week.

Here the emphasis is on obsessions and compulsions based on sexual and religious concerns. Moral concerns that are not explicitly religious in character belong in this category as well. There may be some inherent overlap with the aggressive domain. However, check items in this category if the primary issue concerns sexual, moral, or religious matters.

### Obsessions with sexual content

____ Forbidden or improper sexual thoughts

____ Content involves children or incest

____ Content involves homosexuality

____ Content involves violent sexual acts

### Related compulsions

____ Checking compulsions related to sexual

Obsessions

____ Repeating compulsions related to sexual obsessions

____ Mental rituals related to sexual obsessions

### Avoidance because of sexual obsessions

____ Intentional avoidance of people, places, or things because of any of the above obsessions or compulsions concerning sex

### Obsessions with religious content*

____ Content involves sacrilege or blasphemy

____ Excessive concern with what is morally right or wrong

____ Fear saying certain things

____ Need to tell, ask, or confess things

### Related compulsions

____ Checking or other compulsions related to religious obsessions

____

____ Repeating compulsions related to religious obsessions

____ Mental rituals related to religious obsessions

### Avoidance—religious

____ Intentional avoidance of people, places, or things because of any of the above obsessions or compulsions concerning religious topics

### Other obsessions or compulsions in this category (describe):

_____

_____

### Symptoms in this category were present during the past week?

Yes   No

If yes, complete the next page. If no, skip to next section.

**Severity ratings (past week) for sexual and religious obsessions and related compulsions**

*1. How much of your time is occupied by these obsessions and compulsions?*

0 = **No time at all**.

1 = **Rarely** present during the past week, often not on a daily basis, typically <3 hr/ week.

2 = **Occasionally, >3 hr/week, but <1 hr/day**—occasional intrusion, need to perform compulsions, or avoidance (occurs no >5 times a day).

3 = **Frequently, 1 to 3 hr/day**—frequent intrusion, need to perform compulsions, or avoidance (occurs >8 times a day, but most hours of the day are free of these obsessions, compulsions, and related avoidance).

4 = **Almost always, >3 and up to 8 hr/day**—very frequent intrusion, need to perform compulsions, or avoidance (occurs >8 times a day and occurs during most hours of the day).

5 = **Always, >8 hr/day**—near constant intrusion of obsessions, need to perform compulsions, or avoidance (too numerous to count, and an hour rarely passes without several obsessions, compulsions, and/or avoidance).

*2. How much distress do these obsessions and related compulsions cause?*

0 = **No distress**.

1 = **Minimal**, when symptoms are present, they are minimally distressing.

2 = **Mild**, some clear distress present, but not too disturbing.

3 = **Moderate**, disturbing, but still tolerable.

4 = **Severe**, very disturbing.

5 = **Extreme**, near constant and disabling distress.

*3. How much do these obsessions and related compulsions interfere with your family life, friendships, or ability to perform well at work or at school?*

0 = **No interference**.

1 = **Minimal**, slight interference with social or occupational activities, overall performance not impaired.

2 = **Mild**, some interference with social or occupational activities, overall performance affected to a small degree.

3 = **Moderate**, definite interference with social or occupational performance, but still manageable.

4 = **Severe interference**, causes substantial impairment in social or occupational performance.

5 = **Extreme**, incapacitating interference.

## Checklist of symmetry, ordering, counting, and arranging obsessions and compulsions (past week)

*Checklist*: check once (✓) for any symptoms present during the past week.

This dimension is usually fairly distinctive when present. However, overlaps can occur with other dimensions, particularly when there are concerns about harm or illness. Check these items only if, in your best judgement, the symptoms are best accounted for under this category. Similarly, if you are uncertain about which category best covers the symptoms in question, please indicate your doubts with annotations, and rate the symptoms accordingly in more than one dimension.

*Obsessions*

___ Content involves needing things to be perfect or exact or 'just right'

___ Content involves needing things to be symmetrical or correctly aligned

___ Fear not saying 'just the right thing'

*Compulsions*

___ Checking for own mistakes

___ Ordering and arranging compulsions

___ Compulsions involving touching, tapping, or rubbing

___ Compulsions involving evening up or aligning

Rereading or rewriting compulsions

___ Repeating routine activities

___ Counting compulsions

___ Other mental rituals

*Avoidance*

___ Intentional avoidance of places or things because of these obsessions or compulsions

### Other symptoms in this category (describe):

_____

_____

### Symptoms in this category were present during the past week?

Yes    No

If yes, complete the next page. If no, skip to next section.

**Severity (past week) of symmetry, ordering, counting, and arranging obsessions and compulsions**

*1. How much of your time is occupied by these obsessions and compulsions?*

0 = **No time at all**.

1 = **Rarely** present during the past week, often not on a daily basis, typically <3 hr/week.

2 = **Occasionally, >3 hr/week, but <1 hr/day**—occasional intrusion, need to perform compulsions, or avoidance (occurs no >5 times a day).

3 = **Frequently, 1 to 3 hr/day**—frequent intrusion, need to perform compulsions, or avoidance (occurs >8 times a day, but most hours of the day are free of these obsessions, compulsions, and related avoidance).

4 = **Almost always, >3 and up to 8 hr/day**—very frequent intrusion, need to perform compulsions, or avoidance (occurs >8 times a day and occurs during most hours of the day).

5 = **Always, >8 hr/day**—near constant intrusion of obsessions, need to perform compulsions, or avoidance (too numerous to count, and an hour rarely passes without several obsessions, compulsions, and/or avoidance).

*2. How much distress do these obsessions and related compulsions cause you?*

0 = **No distress**.

1 = **Minimal**, when symptoms are present they are minimally distressing.

2 = **Mild**, some clear distress present, but not too disturbing.

3 = **Moderate**, disturbing but still tolerable.

4 = **Severe**, very disturbing.

5 = **Extreme**, near constant and disabling distress.

*3. How much do these obsessions and related compulsions interfere with your family life, friendships, or ability to perform well at work or at school?*

0 = **No interference**.

1 = **Minimal**, slight interference with social or occupational activities, overall performance not impaired.

2 = **Mild**, some interference with social or occupational activities, overall performance affected to a small degree.

3 = **Moderate**, definite interference with social or occupational performance, but still manageable.

4 = **Severe interference**, causes substantial impairment in social or occupational performance.

5 = **Extreme**, incapacitating interference.

## Checklist of contamination obsessions and cleaning compulsions

**Checklist**: check once (✓) for any symptoms present during the past week.

Again, this category is usually quite distinctive when present, and, in some individuals, it is the only dimension present. Care may be needed to distinguish between aggressive and somatic obsessions. Check only if clear obsessions or compulsions that include contamination content are present.

**Obsessions**

____ Content involves dirt and germs

____ Concerns or disgust with bodily waste or secretions

____ Content involves environmental household contaminants

____ Content involves insects or animals

____ Bothered by sticky substances

____ Content involves worry about becoming ill because of contamination

**Compulsions**

____ Compulsive or ritualized handwashing

____ Repeated cleaning of household items or other inanimate objects

____ Ritualized showering, bathing, or toilet routines

____ Measures taken to prevent contact with household contaminants

____ Mental rituals associated with contamination

**Avoidance**

____ Intentional avoidance of places or things because of these obsessions or compulsions

**Other symptoms in this category (describe):**

_____

_____

**Symptoms in this category were present during the past week?**

Yes    No

If yes, complete the next page. If no, skip to next section.

## Severity (past week) of contamination obsessions and cleaning compulsions

*1. How much of your time is occupied by these obsessions and compulsions?*

0 = **No time at all**.

1 = **Rarely** present during the past week, often not on a daily basis, typically <3 hr/week.

2 = **Occasionally, >3 hr/week, but <1 hr/day**—occasional intrusion, need to perform compulsions, or avoidance (occurs no >5 times a day).

3 = **Frequently, 1 to 3 hr/day**—frequent intrusion, need to perform compulsions, or avoidance (occurs >8 times a day, but most hours of the day are free of these obsessions, compulsions, and related avoidance).

4 = **Almost always, >3 and up to 8 hr/day**—very frequent intrusion, need to perform compulsions, or avoidance (occurs >8 times a day and occurs during most hours of the day).

5 = **Always, >8 hr/day**—near constant intrusion of obsessions, need to perform compulsions, or avoidance (too numerous to count, and an hour rarely passes without several obsessions, compulsions, and/or avoidance).

*2. How much distress do these obsessions and related compulsions cause?*

0 = **No distress**.

1 = **Minimal**, when symptoms are present they are minimally distressing.

2 = **Mild**, some clear distress present, but not too disturbing.

3 = **Moderate**, disturbing, but still tolerable.

4 = **Severe**, very disturbing.

5 = **Extreme**, near constant and disabling distress.

*3. How much do these obsessions and related compulsions interfere with your family life, friendships, or ability to perform well at work or at school?*

0 = **No interference**.

1 = **Minimal**, slight interference with social or occupational activities, overall performance not impaired.

2 = **Mild**, some interference with social or occupational activities, overall performance affected to a small degree.

3 = **Moderate**, definite interference with social or occupational performance, but still manageable.

4 = **Severe interference**, causes substantial impairment in social or occupational performance.

5 = **Extreme**, incapacitating interference.

## Checklist of collecting and hoarding obsessions and compulsions

*Checklist*: check once (✓) for any symptoms present during the past week.

This is a distinctive category that, at times, overlaps with concerns about doing harm. Check only if clear obsessions or compulsions that include collecting and hoarding are present.

### Obsessions

____ Content involves needing to save things

____ Content involves distress over discarding things

____ Unable to decide to throw things away

____ Obsessions about losing things

### Compulsions

____ Hoarding

____ Mental rituals that relate to hoarding

### Avoidance

____ Intentional avoidance of places or things because of these obsessions or compulsions

### Other symptoms in this category (describe):

_____

_____

### Symptoms in this category were present during the past week?

Yes    No

If yes, complete the next page. If no, skip to next section.

## Severity (past week) of collecting and hoarding

*1. How much of your time is occupied by these obsessions and compulsions?*

0 = **No time at all**.

1 = **Rarely** present during the past week, often not on a daily basis, typically <3 hr/ week.

2 = **Occasionally, >3 hr/week, but <1 hr/day**—occasional intrusion, need to perform compulsions, or avoidance (occurs no >5 times a day).

3 = **Frequently, 1 to 3 hr/day**—frequent intrusion, need to perform compulsions, or avoidance (occurs >8 times a day, but most hours of the day are free of these obsessions, compulsions, and related avoidance).

4 = **Almost always, >3 and up to 8 hr/day**—very frequent intrusion, need to perform compulsions, or avoidance (occurs >8 times a day and occurs during most hours of the day).

5 = **Always, >8 hr/day**—near constant intrusion of obsessions, need to perform compulsions, or avoidance (too numerous to count, and an hour rarely passes without several obsessions, compulsions, and/or avoidance).

*2. How much distress do these obsessions and related compulsions cause?*

0 = **No interference**.

1 = **Minimal**, slight interference with social or occupational activities, overall performance not impaired.

2 = **Mild**, some interference with social or occupational activities, overall performance affected to a small degree.

3 = **Moderate**, definite interference with social or occupational performance, but still manageable.

4 = **Severe interference**, causes substantial impairment in social or occupational performance.

5 = **Extreme**, incapacitating interference.

*3. How much do these obsessions and related compulsions interfere with your family life, friendships, or ability to perform well at work or at school?*

0 = **No distress**.

1 = **Minimal**, when symptoms are present, they are minimally distressing.

2 = **Mild**, some clear distress present, but not too disturbing.

3 = **Moderate**, disturbing, but still tolerable.

4 = **Severe**, very disturbing.

5 = **Extreme**, near constant and disabling distress.

## Somatic obsessions and compulsions symptoms

**Checklist**: check once (✓) for any other symptoms present during the past week.

Do not include symptoms related to body dysmorphic disorder or hypochondriasis. In hypochondriasis, subjects believe that they have a serious illness or they are preoccupied with the idea that they do have a serious illness.

| Somatic obsessions | Related compulsions |
|---|---|
| ___ Content involves illness or disease | ___ Checking or other compulsions related to somatic obsessions |
| | ___ Mental rituals, other than checking, related to somatic obsessions |

### Avoidance—somatic obsessions

___ Intentional avoidance of people, places, or things because of any of the above obsessions or compulsions concerning illness or disease

### Other symptoms in this category (describe):

_____

_____

### Symptoms in this category were present during the past week?

Yes    No

If yes, complete the next page. If no, skip to next section.

## Severity (past week) of somatic obsessions and compulsions*

### 1. How much of your time is occupied by these obsessions and compulsions?

0 = **No time at all**.

1 = **Rarely** present during the past week, often not on a daily basis, typically <3 hr/week.

2 = **Occasionally, >3 hr/week, but <1 hr/day**—occasional intrusion, need to perform compulsions, or avoidance (occurs no >5 times a day).

3 = **Frequently, 1 to 3 hr/day**—frequent intrusion, need to perform compulsions, or avoidance (occurs >8 times a day, but most hours of the day are free of these obsessions, compulsions, and related avoidance).

4 = **Almost always, >3 and up to 8 hr/day**—very frequent intrusion, need to perform compulsions, or avoidance (occurs >8 times a day and occurs during most hours of the day).

5 = **Always, >8 hr/day**—near constant intrusion of obsessions, need to perform compulsions, or avoidance (too numerous to count, and an hour rarely passes without several obsessions, compulsions, and/or avoidance).

### 2. How much distress do these obsessions and related compulsions cause?

0 = **No distress**.

1 = **Minimal**, when symptoms are present, they are minimally distressing.

2 = **Mild**, some clear distress present, but not too disturbing.

3 = **Moderate**, disturbing, but still tolerable.

4 = **Severe**, very disturbing.

5 = **Extreme**, near constant and disabling distress.

### 3. How much do these obsessions and related compulsions interfere with your family life, friendships, or ability to perform well at work or at school?

0 = **No interference**.

1 = **Minimal**, slight interference with social or occupational activities, overall performance not impaired.

2 = **Mild**, some interference with social or occupational activities, overall performance affected to a small degree.

3 = **Moderate**, definite interference with social or occupational performance, but still manageable.

4 = **Severe interference**, causes substantial impairment in social or occupational performance.

5 = **Extreme**, incapacitating interference.

131

# Miscellaneous symptoms

**Checklist**: check once (✓) for any other symptoms present during the past week.

*Miscellaneous obsessions*

| | |
|---|---|
| ___ | Superstitious fears |
| ___ | Luck or unlucky numbers |
| ___ | Colours with special significance |
| ___ | Intrusive nonsense sounds, words, or music |
| ___ | Intrusive (non-violent) images |
| ___ | Need to know or remember certain things |

*Compulsions*

| | |
|---|---|
| ___ | Superstitious behaviour |
| ___ | Related compulsions |
| ___ | Related compulsions |
| ___ | Related compulsions |
| ___ | Related compulsions |
| ___ | Excessive list making |
| ___ | Compulsions are: knowing, remembering |
| ___ | Obsessive slowness |

*Avoidance associated with miscellaneous obsessions and compulsions*

___  Intentional avoidance of places or things because of these obsessions or compulsions

*Other symptoms in this category (describe):*

_____

_____

*Symptoms in this category were present during the past week?*

Yes   No

If yes, complete the next page. If no, skip to next section.

## Severity (past week) of miscellaneous obsessions and compulsions*

*1. How much of your time is occupied by these obsessions and compulsions?*

0 = **No time at all**.

1 = **Rarely** present during the past week, often not on a daily basis, typically <3 hr/week.

2 = **Occasionally, >3 hr/week, but <1 hr/day**—occasional intrusion, need to perform compulsions, or avoidance (occurs no >5 times a day).

3 = **Frequently, 1 to 3 hr/day**—frequent intrusion, need to perform compulsions, or avoidance (occurs >8 times a day, but most hours of the day are free of these obsessions, compulsions, and related avoidance).

4 = **Almost always, >3 and up to 8 hr/day**—very frequent intrusion, need to perform compulsions, or avoidance (occurs >8 times a day and occurs during most hours of the day).

5 = **Always, >8 hr/day**—near constant intrusion of obsessions, need to perform compulsions, or avoidance (too numerous to count, and an hour rarely passes without several obsessions, compulsions, and/or avoidance).

*2. How much distress do these obsessions and related compulsions cause?*

0 = **No distress**.

1 = **Minimal**, when symptoms are present, they are minimally distressing.

2 = **Mild**, some clear distress present, but not too disturbing.

3 = **Moderate**, disturbing, but still tolerable.

4 = **Severe**, very disturbing.

5 = **Extreme**, near constant and disabling distress.

*3. How much do these obsessions and related compulsions interfere with your family life, friendships, or ability to perform well at work or at school?*

0 = **No interference**.

1 = **Minimal**, slight interference with social or occupational activities, overall performance not impaired.

2 = **Mild**, some interference with social or occupational activities, overall performance affected to a small degree.

3 = **Moderate**, definite interference with social or occupational performance, but still manageable.

4 = **Severe interference**, causes substantial impairment in social or occupational performance.

5 = **Extreme**, incapacitating interference.

* Just include the obsessions and compulsions listed under 'Miscellaneous symptoms' in making these severity ratings.

# Global obsessive–compulsive symptom severity

*Indicate your best judgement concerning which symptom categories are present.* Review with the patient how well their obsessions and compulsions fit within a given symptom category: 2 = clearly present and symptoms are readily understood in terms of a given symptom dimension; 1 = might be present, but significant uncertainty exists such that their symptoms are not readily understood in terms of a given symptom dimension; 0 = symptoms within a given dimension were absent or 'probably absent' during the past week.

_____  Aggressive obsessions and related compulsions

_____  Sexual and religious obsessions and related compulsions

_____  Symmetry, ordering, counting, and arranging obsessions and compulsions

_____  Contamination obsessions and cleaning compulsions

_____  Collecting and hoarding obsessions and compulsions

_____  Somatic obsessions and compulsions

_____  Miscellaneous obsessions and compulsions

**Rank order the symptom categories by severity for the past week.** 1 = most severe, 2 = next most severe, and so on. Please mark each category. If symptoms were absent during the past week, place a '0' in the space provided.

_____  Aggressive obsessions and related compulsions

_____  Sexual and religious obsessions and related compulsions

_____  Symmetry, ordering, counting, and arranging obsessions and compulsions

_____  Contamination obsessions and cleaning compulsions

_____  Collecting and hoarding

_____  Somatic obsessions and compulsions

_____  Miscellaneous obsessions and compulsions

**List the patient's most prominent obsessive–compulsive symptoms:**

1. _____

2. _____

3. _____

*What is the worst thing that the patient worries will happen if she/he did not respond to obsessive thoughts or urges to perform compulsions or rituals? Please describe:*

_____

_____

_____

_____

_____

*How certain is the patient that this feared consequence is reasonable and will actually occur?*

- 0 = Certain that the feared consequence will not happen
- 1 = Mostly certain that the feared consequence will not happen
- 2 = Unsure whether or not the feared consequence will or won't happen
- 3 = Mostly certain that the feared consequence will happen
- 4 = Certain that the feared consequence will happen

*Finally review all obsessive–compulsive symptoms endorsed as occurring during the past week* (excluding 'other' symptoms judged not to be bona fide obsessive–compulsive symptoms), and make a global severity rating for the past week using the ordinal scales on the next page, and complete the score sheet.

*Reliability of informant(s)* Excellent = 0   Good = 1   Fair = 2   Poor = 3

## Global severity obsessions and compulsions (past week)

*1. How much of your time is occupied by these obsessions and compulsions?*

0 = **No time at all**.

1 = **Rarely** present during the past week, often not on a daily basis, typically <3 hr/ week.

2 = **Occasionally, >3 hr/week, but <1 hr/day**—occasional intrusion, need to perform compulsions, or avoidance (occurs no >5 times a day).

3 = **Frequently, 1 to 3 hr/day**—frequent intrusion, need to perform compulsions, or avoidance (occurs >8 times a day, but most hours of the day are free of these obsessions, compulsions, and related avoidance).

4 = **Almost always, >3 and up to 8 hr/day**—very frequent intrusion, need to perform compulsions, or avoidance (occurs >8 times a day and occurs during most hours of the day).

5 = **Always, >8 hr/day**—near constant intrusion of obsessions, need to perform compulsions, or avoidance (too numerous to count, and an hour rarely passes without several obsessions, compulsions, and/or avoidance).

*2. How much distress do these obsessions and related compulsions cause?*

0 = **No interference**.

1 = **Minimal**, slight interference with social or occupational activities, overall performance not impaired.

2 = **Mild**, some interference with social or occupational activities, overall performance affected to a small degree.

3 = **Moderate**, definite interference with social or occupational performance, but still manageable.

4 = **Severe interference**, causes substantial impairment in social or occupational performance.

5 = **Extreme**, incapacitating interference.

*3. How much do these obsessions and related compulsions interfere with your family life, friendships, or ability to perform well at work or at school?*

0 = **No distress**.

1 = **Minimal**, when symptoms are present, they are minimally distressing.

2 = **Mild**, some clear distress present, but not too disturbing.

3 = **Moderate**, disturbing, but still tolerable.

4 = **Severe**, very disturbing.

5 = **Extreme**, near constant and disabling distress.

## DY-BOCS score sheet

Patient's name _____

Today's date: ___ / ___ / ___
              mm  dd  yy

Clinician _____

### 1. DY-BOCS clinician severity ratings by symptom category for the past week

| Symptom category | Time (0–5) | Interference (0–5) | Distress (0–5) | Total (0–5) |
|---|---|---|---|---|
| Aggressive | | | | |
| Sexual and religious | | | | |
| Symmetry, ordering, counting, and arranging | | | | |
| Contamination and cleaning | | | | |
| Hoarding and collecting | | | | |
| Somatic | | | | |
| Miscellaneous | | | | |

### 2. DY-DOCS global severity ratings for the past week

| | Time (0–5) | Interference (0–5) | Distress (0–5) | Total (0–5) |
|---|---|---|---|---|
| All obsessions and compulsions | | | | |

Time required to complete the ratings _____ minutes

Reproduced with permission from Dr James Leckman

# Obsessive–compulsive spectrum symptoms

_____ *Other somatic obsessions\**

_____ Content involves bodily appearance

_____ Content involves food or eating

_____ Content concerns the urge to pluck hair

_____ Content concerns the urge to pick skin

_____ *Related compulsions*

_____ Related grooming compulsions

_____ Related dressing compulsions

_____ Related eating habits

_____ Related compulsions related to physical exercise

_____ Trichotillomania

_____ Skin picking

*Obsessions related to separation or union\**

_____ Concerns about being separated from a close family member

_____ Concerns about becoming or being too much like another person

*Compulsions*

_____ Compulsions to prevent the loss of a close family member

_____ Related compulsions

*Tic-related obsessions\**

_____ Staring rituals

_____ Urge to repeat something you heard

\* As in the original Y-BOCS, do not include these obsessions and compulsions in the severity ratings. Specialized rated instruments should be employed to rate separation anxiety disorder, tic disorders, eating disorders, body dysmorphic disorder, and trichotillomania. They are included here to document obsessive-compulsive spectrum symptoms for research purposes.

# Clinical Global Impression (CGI)

The Clinical Global Impression (CGI) is a brief 3-item clinician-rated scale that assesses illness severity, improvement/change, and response to treatment. The illness severity and improvement items are more frequently used by clinicians and researchers than the therapeutic response section, and, for that reason, only the former have been reproduced in this volume.

## Reference

Guy W (1976). CGI Clinical global impressions. In: *Early Clinical Drug Evaluation Program (ECDEU) assessment manual for psychopharmacology* (revised DHEW Publ No ADM 76–338). Rockville, MD: US Department of Health, Education and Welfare, National Institute of Mental Health, pp. 217–22.

# Clinical Global Impression Scale for Severity

The rating considers the clinician's entire experience with the disorder under investigation and the severity of that condition at the current time. Note that it is the severity of the particular condition that is rated, and not psychiatric illness generally.

Routine clinical CGI(s) differs from the CGI(s) scale usually used for research by 1 point.

Routine clinical CGI(s) is coded on a 0 to 6 scale as follows:

0 = not ill

1 = borderline ill

2 = mildly ill

3 = moderately ill

4 = markedly ill

5 = severely ill

6 = among the most extremely ill

x = not assessed

Research CGI(s) is coded on a 0 to 7 scale as follows:

0 = not assessed

1 = normal, not ill

2 = borderline ill

3 = mildly ill

4 = moderately ill

5 = markedly ill

6 = severely ill

7 = among the most extremely ill

# Clinical Global Impression Scale for Improvement

The rating considers the degree of change since the start of the current treatment plan. The rating does not consider whether the improvement is related to therapy or not.

Routine clinical CGI(i) is coded as follows:

+3 = very much improved

+2 = much improved

+1 = minimally improved

0 = unchanged

−1 = minimally worse

−2 = much worse

−3 = very much worse

x = not assessed

Research CGI(i) is coded as follows:

0 = not assessed

1 = very much improved

2 = much improved

3 = minimally improved

4 = unchanged

5 = minimally worse

6 = much worse

7 = very much worse

The CGI is available in the public domain.

# Index

141